3 9077 04107311 8

D1502508

ummond, Edward H.

**Overcoming anxie-
ty without tran-
quilizers**

$5.95

DUE DATE

INTRODUCTION

As I finished writing this book, I treated a man who suffered from anxiety for many years and depended on Ativan, a benzodiazepine, to bring him some measure of relief. He was divorced, unemployed, and deeply discouraged about his life. Because of his physical appearance and his difficulties, he reminded me of a patient I had seen during my training in psychiatry in 1983. Although the cases were similar, my recommendations for treatment were vastly different because of all that I had learned in the intervening years.

My earlier patient was dependent on Xanax, another benzodiazepine. He suffered from intense panic attacks in public, which led him to restrict himself from going out of his apartment. He was able to get out with the aid of the Xanax, but he began each day with feelings of dread. At that time, Xanax was being aggressively marketed for panic attacks, and this poor man felt that he couldn't survive without it. I believed him—which I have gradually learned was a big mistake—and continued to prescribe it for him. Besides using Xanax, we tried to decrease his anxiety by working on his problems in psychotherapy. He also forced himself to go out of the house and into public places several times a week in the hope that regular practice would make venturing out easier. He felt a little better as we continued our work together. No matter what we did, however, he experienced intense anxiety whenever he went more than a few hours without his Xanax. We parted amicably when I finished my training and left the area, but I always felt that something wasn't right. At the time, I was unable to articulate what gave rise to my uneasiness.

1

When I went out into practice, I found that most patients with anxiety disorders, depression, schizophrenia, and bipolar disorder derived significant benefit from medications, psychotherapy, or both. As I continued to practice, however, I gradually saw that there was one group of people who didn't seem to get better—people who suffered from chronic anxiety and who took benzodiazepines such as Valium, Xanax, Ativan, or Klonopin for relief.

My search to find ways to help people with chronic anxiety who depended on these drugs led me to question the understanding of anxiety and the methods that doctors use to treat it. I have come to see that benzodiazepines have profoundly negative effects on a person's life, and that the only way to help a patient overcome chronic anxiety is to help him or her get off them. This understanding didn't come all at once; different patients helped me to see different aspects of the issues involved. As a result, the overall approach that I've developed came together gradually.

The knowledge that I've gained during this search led me to recommend a very different treatment to the patient who walked through my office door this year compared to what I offered fifteen years ago. I no longer believed that anyone had to go through life as a victim of anxiety, and I knew that this man could do better. I didn't want to prescribe a habit-forming benzodiazepine like Ativan that could also impair his memory and coordination. I wanted him to learn to manage his anxiety in ways that would strengthen his sense of himself and bolster his confidence—not give him a pill whose message was that he couldn't manage life. I knew that he could reclaim his life from the clutches of anxiety and a dependency on Ativan and learn to enjoy himself. I knew it wouldn't be easy, but I knew we could be successful.

He was doubtful when I said he needed to come off what he perceived to be his only aid. Although I tried to be as gentle and supportive as I could, he looked at me with dislike and anger. An unpleasant moment for us both. When we looked at each other, both feeling uncomfortable, I wished I *could* offer him (and everyone else) an easy cure. Although it's only too easy to prescribe benzos, unfortunately they're no cure—they're a recipe for disaster. Offering a difficult cure was the best I could do.

Because so many patients have expressed their deepest thanks to me when they are finally off their pills and have reclaimed their lives, I acknowledged his skepticism, hostility, and anger but did not alter my stance. Instead, I focused on the benefits of a life without medication, in which he felt good about himself and what he was doing, and in which *he* was in control, not a pill. I tried to help him see that his life had become narrowed and unsatisfying because of the way that he chose to manage anxiety, i.e., taking a pill. I held forth the hope that his relationships, work, and other interests could be far more satisfying if he took the difficult step of trying a new way of managing his anxiety.

After preparing for some weeks with ways that I discuss in the book, we cut his daily Ativan dose by about ten percent. He tolerated the decrease by learning to focus directly on his anxiety, rather than running from it at all costs. He learned other ways of managing his anxiety besides reaching for a pill. As he mastered some new techniques, he felt increasingly confident about his ability to handle anxiety and increasingly hopeful that he would be able to stop the Ativan entirely. Each month we made another small decrease in his daily dosage. As he began to feel more confident, he stopped spending his energy managing anxiety. He began to pay more and more attention to his life and how to make it more satisfying. He began to date again. He obtained work that was below his potential but that offered the opportunity for advancement. His preoccupation with anxiety and craving for Ativan receded.

When we got down to stopping the final dose he knew that his desire for the medication was because he had become used to taking it, not because his body needed it. With feelings of excitement and trepidation, he stopped taking it. He was relieved, excited, and proud that he accomplished his goal of stopping the pills without feeling overwhelmed with anxiety. He vowed never to take another one.

You may think that stopping your benzodiazepine is beyond your capability. It isn't. I know because I have helped hundreds of people do it. It will be one of the hardest tasks you will ever undertake, but if you follow the step-by-step process I describe in the book, you can stop taking benzodiazepines, master your anxiety, and reclaim your life.

I'm indebted to the patients who shared their thoughts, feelings, and experiences with me and helped me to see the devastation caused by a dependency on benzodiazepines. I have changed their names and altered the descriptions of their experiences in order to protect their confidentiality. The case histories presented

in this book are fictional composites based on my professional experience in treating anxiety disorders. The particular brand names
of benzodiazepines mentioned in the context of the case histories
are for purposes of illustrating the conditions that I have found are
common to the use of benzodiazepine drugs. I do not suggest that
each person who takes a particular drug referenced in the case histories will experience the same effects or will have the same results
if they discontinue use. I write this book in gratitude to my patients
and in hope that other people who are dependent on benzodiazepines for the relief of chronic anxiety can use this knowledge to
end their destructive dependency and take charge of their lives.

EDWARD H. DRUMMOND, M.D.

Part ♦ One

ANXIETY AND BENZOS

"For the relief of anxiety"—Xanax. "Second to none; unsurpassed efficacy; The one you know best, the best one to know"—Valium. "It does effectively relieve anxiety"—Ativan. "Distinctive, patient preferred, effective not overpowering; anxioselective"—Tranxene.

**—Advertisements for benzodiazepines
in the *American Journal of Psychiatry***

♦

Isn't it the universal opinion that our town is a healthy spot? Quite an unusually healthy spot, in fact,—a place that deserves to be recommended in the warmest possible manner. . . . We have been recommending it and praising it. . . . And the baths—we have called them the "main artery of the town's life-blood," the "nerve-center of our town" and the devil knows what else. Well, do you know what they really are, these great, splendid, much praised baths, that have cost so much money—do you know what they are? The whole place is a pesthouse.

**—Henrik Ibsen
*An Enemy of the People***

· 1 ·

THE BENZO BLUES

An otherwise well young woman comes to an emergency room with a pounding heart and shortness of breath. She is reassured that she has suffered a panic attack, not a heart attack, and is given Ativan, which quickly calms her down. Five years later, she is still taking Ativan daily, despite periodic attempts to get off it, and is constantly worried about when she will have her next panic attack. A woman in her seventies is anxious about her medical problems

TABLE 1

BENZODIAZEPINES

GENERIC	BRAND NAME
alprazolam	Xanax
chlordiazepoxide	Librium
clonazepam	Klonopin
clorazepate	Tranxene
diazepam	Valium
flurazepam	Dalmane
lorazepam	Ativan
oxazepam	Serax
quazepam	Doral
temazepam	Restoril
triazolam	Halcion

and is given Serax to help her relax. She starts to take it regularly and becomes even more anxious and incapacitated as the months go by. A forty-year-old man with a pregnant wife has difficulty sleeping and is prescribed Klonopin. Two years later he's constantly anxious in spite of using Klonopin and barely able to work. A forty-nine-year-old woman develops anxiety and insomnia after her husband dies and is prescribed Xanax and Restoril. Three years later she's still on them. She's given up most of the activities she's previously enjoyed and is a shell of her former self.

What these people have in common is a syndrome that I've come to call the "Benzo Blues"—a serious but solvable problem that has arisen with the overselling and overprescription of benzodiazepines, "benzos" for short. Benzodiazepines are taken by tens of millions of people each year in the United States to suppress the symptoms of anxiety and relieve insomnia. Most people take them only for a few days or weeks to get them through a crisis situation, but almost four million people in the United States, and millions more in other countries, end up taking them every day for years. Unfortunately, people who take the drugs for more than a few weeks often become physically and psychologically dependent on them and then find themselves unable to move on in their lives and solve the problems that are leading them to be anxious. In other words, they have the "Benzo Blues." What is most distressing is that instead of solving or curing the problems of anxiety, their regular use actually promotes and maintains chronic anxiety, interferes with the pursuit of treatment that is truly effective, and leads to unnecessary restrictions in the lives of people who take them. This is a worldwide scandal in which the interests of society, drug companies, third-party payment organizations such as insurance companies and HMOs, doctors, patients, and the effects of the drugs themselves combine to keep patients dependent.

The extensive use of benzodiazepines and other psychiatric drugs, such as Prozac for depression, Ritalin for attention deficit disorder, and lithium for bipolar disorder, has been a central part of the "biological revolution" that is supposedly providing relief for all forms of psychiatric distress. This revolution has dramatically transformed the field of mental health, especially the practice of psychiatry. Drugs, rather than talk or other forms of therapy, have become the main form of treatment. And although substantial numbers of people have gotten significant relief, many problems associated with drug use have been largely ignored. The widespread and prolonged use of benzodiazepines for anxiety is especially troubling because it has been known since their development in the fifties and early sixties that they are habit-forming. Many patients and doctors minimize the problem of addiction, however, focusing instead on the relief the drugs provide to people in battling anxiety.

For some years I thought that the problems of people who took benzodiazepines were due principally to their circumstances and their anxiety. I continued to prescribe the benzodiazepines, even though I disliked doing so because I knew that they were habit-forming. I began to question, though, the understanding of anxiety offered by the psychiatric profession and the usefulness of the treatments that I had been taught.

I began to see that when people take benzodiazepines because they are anxious they come to rely on the drugs as their only aid in the daily struggle to tolerate the symptoms of anxiety. They avoid activities that might lead them to be anxious but also give up pursuits that would be enjoyable for them. They feel beaten down in their lives. Let's look at four people with anxiety who take these drugs.

Susan was twenty-nine when she came to see me. A bright, attractive single woman, she worked as a computer sales representative for a company that was expanding rapidly. "I've had panic attacks for years, but I've been able to function okay as long as I took my Ativan. Now, however, I've been offered a new position that would require me to fly all over the country. I'd like to take the new job, but I'm terrified of flying and don't think I can do it. It's not that I'd mind the travel; in fact, I'd like to see different places. I don't know why, but I don't think I could step on a plane now if you pointed a gun to my head."

"How long have you been anxious?" I asked.

"I was fine until I was twenty-four. I'll never forget that day. I was driving with my boyfriend to a restaurant when I had my first panic attack. Of course, I didn't know what it was at the time. I just knew I couldn't breathe, my heart was pounding, and I thought I was going to die of a heart attack. I almost threw up in the car when we went to the emergency room. Then we had to wait for what seemed like hours until I had a cardiogram. It was normal, luckily, but I didn't really calm down until the doctor gave me a shot of Ativan."

"Panic attacks can be one of the most unpleasant experiences in a person's life," I said, "and yours sound really terrible. If I were in your shoes I would never want to have another one."

"The weird thing is that they just seem to come out of the blue," Susan said. "There doesn't seem to be any reason for them. I've seen three doctors over the years and therapists. I've tried those breathing exercises but nothing has helped me the way that Ativan has. I still have them, but they happen much less often now. I've tried to get off the Ativan a couple of times, but the panic attacks start right up again so I go back on it. I wish I didn't have to depend on the medication, but my anxiety is just terrible."

"It seems that even when you're not having a panic attack, you're worried about having another one. Do you avoid certain activities in order to minimize the chance you might have another one?"

"I used to avoid going to stores and malls—anyplace where I'd be in a crowd or feel that I couldn't get out. I still avoid being a passenger in a car, although I can drive okay. I like to be the one in control, I guess. At least that's what my boyfriend says," she said with a smile. "But that's really why I'm here. I've never flown before—I've always been able to get around it somehow—but I'll have to if I take this new job. I turned it down at first, but my boss pestered me until I told him what I was worried about. He said he'd keep the offer on the table for a few more weeks. He talked me into seeing a psychiatrist."

Like many people with panic attacks, Susan was constantly on the alert for the next one. Although she thought the pills helped her, we will see that they actually hinder her ability to overcome panic attacks when we look at her difficulties in more detail.

Janet was seventy-five when her internist referred her to me. Initially, she didn't want to come because she didn't like the idea of seeing a psychiatrist, but she kept the appointment that he made for her.

"I've been seeing Dr. Crandal for years," she said. "I don't really know why he sent me to see you. I don't want to see a psychiatrist. I've got colitis, high blood pressure, and allergies, but Dr. Crandal has always taken perfectly good care of me. I'm on a number of medications including sulfasalazine, Dyazide, Inderal, cimetidine for stomach acid, Fiorinal when I need it for headaches, which seems to be all the time now, and Serax for my nerves. Sometimes I take a Restoril if I don't sleep too well. I had a bout of colitis recently; in fact, I just got out of the hospital after I lost almost twenty pounds."

"Did Dr. Crandal ever find out why you had a flare-up of your colitis?" I asked, knowing that stress can often make it worse.

"No, but I've had these flare-ups all my life, although they've been more frequent ever since I went through the change of life. It's partly my nerves, I know that, but I've always been a nervous person. That's why he gives me the Serax; it calms me right down. Lately I've been so worried about this colitis, though, that even the Serax doesn't seem to be helping as much as it usually does. I've been worried about my health, I have to admit it. I'm an independent kind of person, and I don't like to be sick. When I grew up during the Depression, I took care of my brothers and sisters so that my mother could go to work. It wasn't easy, but I learned I had to take care of myself. I gave some things up in my life, we all did, but we were as happy as any family could be. That's what's so hard for me now—I'm just not used to being sick. There are times it's got me so upset I even cry."

"When did things start to go bad for you?" I asked.

"I was all right up until a couple of years ago. Then Dr. Crandal discovered I had high blood pressure. I didn't want to take any of his pills until he scared me by telling me that I might have a stroke. I never really thought about death much—I was always the one taking care of other people and not thinking too much about myself. But then I began to be anxious all the time. I wasn't afraid of anything in particular, like having a stroke or that I'd choke on my food and no one would be around to save me; it's just that I felt anxious all the time. I couldn't sit still. The Serax helped me at first. I could still drive and get around and see my brothers and sisters. But then I had a car accident and I felt that I shouldn't drive anymore. So I stopped.

"My family visits me now instead of the other way around. I never married and I don't have any children of my own, but I'm the third of eleven kids and I've still got most of my siblings and a pile of nieces and nephews. Even though I see them almost as much, though, it's just not the same."

"What's different?" I asked.

"I'm not the one helping them. They're all helping me instead. Things have gotten all turned around somehow, and I'm a mess. I know I told you that I didn't want to see a psychiatrist, but that's because I'm used to standing on my own. I know I need help. What can you do?"

There was actually a great deal that could be done for Janet, as we'll see.

Jim had been on Klonopin for two years when he first came to me. He was forty-two, married with two young children, and he worked as an assembler at a glass manufacturing company. Jim's family doctor had been prescribing Klonopin for anxiety but felt Jim needed counseling because the anxiety had been going on for two years and was getting worse. The last time he saw his doctor, Jim burst into tears.

"I don't know what's going on, Doc. Everything should be going great—the problem is me. I've been having problems at work because of anxiety for a while. Lately it seems like I can't do my job anymore. I work with molds, and the sizes have to be exact. The day before I saw my doctor, I had to leave work because I was so anxious I couldn't calm down enough to make the measurements properly. I kept thinking that I might make a mistake, and I got so worried about it I finally took the rest of the day off.

"I can't relax, I don't enjoy anything, I don't sleep very well, so I'm irritable all the time. I yell at my wife and kid and even at my baby, which I know is ridiculous, and I feel guilty about it. My wife and I have been married for twelve years, and she's been really great in spite of how I've been, but even she's getting sick of it."

"When did you first start having problems?" I asked.

"I did fine until my wife got pregnant—but it wasn't that I was upset about the pregnancy. We tried to have kids for years before we finally got lucky. I was dying to have kids. I don't know what it was at the time, but it seemed like I just couldn't get to sleep. At first I just took the Klonopin a couple of days a week. As the pregnancy continued, though, I got anxious during the day at work. I would lose my sense of concentration. I started making mistakes. I stopped hanging out with my friends during lunch so I could finish my work. Then I stopped hanging out with them at all because I was too tense to have fun with them.

"When the baby was born, my wife stopped working and our income dropped. We had planned for this and had savings, but I couldn't stop worrying."

"You felt like everything was on your shoulders now that your wife wasn't working and you had a baby?"

"Yes. I got more anxious and started taking the Klonopin during the day to relax. I didn't take it every day at first, but it seemed like when I didn't take it I was just barely holding on. I felt especially nervous around the baby. It seemed like I just couldn't be comfortable around him. Then my wife got pregnant again. We were both excited about the second pregnancy, but I got even more anxious. I always said I'd never let my kids down the way my father let me down. He died when I was only eight."

"So you feel that you're getting worse, not better. And you also feel the need to take the Klonopin regularly because even though you're still anxious, it seems to help you get through the day."

"That's right."

As many people do when they experience anxiety for an extended period of time, Jim felt helpless and overwhelmed. As we'll see, he learned that his hopelessness was unwarranted and that he could overcome his anxiety and benzodiazepine dependency.

Marilyn told me that she had been "worrying too much" since the death of her husband three years earlier. They had been married for almost thirty years when he died of a heart attack while shoveling snow. "I feel like I've been unable to move on. I know I'll never forget Dave or stop loving him, but my life has come to a standstill. We used to be really active together, but now I hardly do anything. That's why my son insisted that I come in to see you. He thinks I need help."

"Losing a husband of thirty years is difficult for anybody," I said. "No one would find it easy to start up a new life. How was it for you at first?"

"I was shocked because Dave had never been sick. He was always the strong one. I always knew I leaned on him, but I never realized how much until he died. It wasn't so much the things Dave did that I missed. It was the day-to-day sharing, waking up together, doing the dishes. We would trade off who did the dishes, but the other person would always sit and talk. Dave was always full of opinions about politics, and we liked to watch the news before we went to bed. After he died, I got so I couldn't sleep. My doctor gave me some Dalmane to help me fall asleep more easily.

"I also take Xanax during the day whenever my nerves act up. Sometimes I just can't sit still, and I need something to calm me down. I find it difficult to concentrate and I can't relax. The only thing that helps me is the Xanax. As soon as I take it, I feel a little better, more relaxed. Without the Xanax I don't know where I'd be.

"I'm not able to handle the things that were an important part of my life before. I've given up our house because there were too many things to worry about. Not just the bills, but the repairs that are always needed and the upkeep on the yard and the garden. I never drove very much—Dave always drove when we went out—but now I've given up my car, too. I used to enjoy many of the activities at my church, but now I only go when my daughter takes me."

"It seems like you've given up some of the things you do because you feel you can't handle them," I commented. "Do you think you really are incapable of managing them?"

"I don't know if I am or not," Marilyn answered, "but I know I'm too afraid to try. I just feel a weight on my shoulders that is too heavy for me to bear."

Marilyn felt unable to cope with life itself, not just with anxiety. We'll return to her story and to the stories of others throughout this book. We'll see how these people developed their anxiety, what the different kinds of anxiety are, what causes anxiety, and, most important, how they stopped taking the medication and took charge of their lives again.

ANXIETY

Susan, Janet, Jim, and Marilyn all experience intense anxiety and use benzodiazepines to help them tolerate the symptoms. But just what is anxiety? Don't we all get it sometimes? Are there different kinds?

Anxiety is the name given to a constellation of thoughts, feelings, physical sensations, and behaviors that we experience when we are worried about something. "Normal" anxiety is something we all experience in stressful situations that occur in everyday life.

Anxiety may develop over small concerns such as getting to an appointment on time, or whether we will accomplish some necessary task. Larger issues can include starting a new job, paying bills, meeting with the boss, proposing marriage, or going through with the wedding. We refer to these feelings as the "willies," the "jitters," or as "nerves." If we are worried about a specific event such as taking a test or going to a job interview, the anxious feelings may intensify and even include some physical sensations such as trembling, dry mouth, sweaty palms, queasy stomach, or diarrhea. It's important to recognize that although anxiety isn't pleasant, it's not necessarily a bad thing; in fact, it helps us to be prepared for upcoming life events. Goaded by the sensations of normal anxiety, we study for exams, pay our taxes on time, and practice for our driving tests.

The medical and psychiatric professions have generally used the term "pathological" to describe anxiety when it has intensified out of proportion to the situation or lasts beyond the event or situation that appears to trigger it. The problem is then referred to as an "anxiety disorder." People with pathological anxiety may experience anxiety in conjunction with what appear to be harmless activities. For example, Susan had her first "anxiety attack," sometimes called a "panic attack," when she was on her way to a restaurant. Unlike those of normal anxiety, the symptoms of pathological anxiety are severe enough that they actually interfere with a person's ability to function. Such symptoms generally include intensely unpleasant physical sensations such as shortness of breath, chest pain, and restlessness, as well as difficulty concentrating and insomnia.

Over the years, opinions about the causes and nature of pathological anxiety have varied. One widely held view is that it is an exceedingly unpleasant experience that strikes a person because of a chemical imbalance. This view is furthered by forms of anxiety, such as obsessive-compulsive disorder and panic disorder, that appear to be caused at least in part by a biological abnormality, though none has been found thus far. Most people with pathological anxiety, however, including many who suffer with panic disorder, have experienced traumatic situations earlier in their life. Sometimes the trauma is recent. Other times it occurred during childhood, and the aftereffects have festered beneath the surface for many years.

The central role that trauma plays in the creation of anxiety has been minimized and even ignored during the years of the so-called biological revolution. As a result, clinicians' recommendations have slanted toward quick solutions like medications and away from the more complex treatment that would be needed to help a person come to terms with past experiences. The narrow biological viewpoint has shortchanged millions of people because they do not receive any treatment that addresses their traumatic experiences.

One in ten people in the United States will experience an anxiety disorder that will cause impairment in functioning at some point in their lives. The serious nature of anxiety disorders is often minimized, both by people who have one and by those around them. Many people feel that those who suffer anxiety should just "get over it." Unfortunately, although some people experience pathological anxiety for only a brief period, all too many people experience disabling symptoms for many years. These people experience what is known as chronic anxiety. As the symptoms persist, sufferers of chronic anxiety lose hope that their symptoms will ever go away and believe they will need to tolerate them as an ever present part of their life. They continue to be very troubled by their symptoms and will do whatever they can to minimize and avoid them. As a result, many become dependent on benzodiazepines, even though other treatment methods are far more effective for chronic anxiety.

BENZODIAZEPINES

The first benzodiazepine released was Librium, in 1960, and Valium appeared three years later. It appeared that this class of drugs shared none of problems associated with previous tranquilizers such as barbiturates. Sedation at normal doses was minimal. Dependence on them, though recognized early on as a possibility, was thought to occur only at high dosages and then only rarely. Death from overdosage was rare.

The apparent safety of the first benzodiazepines led to the synthesis of over three thousand of them, although only thirty-five or so have been marketed. They virtually replaced the other tranquilizers within ten years. In 1965 thirty million prescriptions were written for them. By 1973 the total was up to eighty-seven million.[1] Today, two-thirds of all benzodiazepine prescriptions are written by general practitioners, family practitioners, and internists, with most of the rest written by psychiatrists. In any given year, ten percent of the population in the United States is given a prescription for them.

Almost as soon as they were first synthesized clinically, it became apparent that they could induce a withdrawal reaction similar to narcotics and barbiturates. The first paper documenting the effects appeared in 1961 and reported that patients who were given Librium for one to seven months in the rather high dosage range of 100 to 600 milligrams per day experienced withdrawal symptoms that included epileptic convulsions.[2] Malcolm Lader, M.D., an English physician who has studied the effects of benzodiazepines for more than twenty years, published a series of articles in the eighties and nineties demonstrating that physical dependence can occur within two to three weeks and certainly within four months when people take this class of drug at usual therapeutic ranges.[3]

They are characteristically used to treat anxiety for four different periods of time: single dose, short term, extended, and chronic. These periods are defined in part by time, but also for the purpose of their use. A single dose is commonly employed when people must participate in an activity, such as a plane ride or funeral, that is over in a few hours. Short-term use extends up until physical dependence sets in—approximately four weeks. Extended use occurs for longer than one month. Physical dependence occurs, but the use ends when the situation that is leading to the anxiety resolves. Extended use can occur in the context of the stress of divorce, illness of a family member, unemployment, or court cases. Chronic use occurs when people have no plan or intention to stop their use no matter what happens. Researchers generally consider continuous use longer than one year as chronic.

Many people slide from brief or extended use into chronic use without any specific intention to do so. A 1979 survey of drug use in the United States found that 1.65 percent of the population, almost four million people, had been using benzodiazepines daily for more than one year.[4] About one-third had been taking them for more than three years and another third for more than seven years. Their popularity is not confined to the United States: The frequency of daily use longer than one year in Chile is 5.9 percent, Belgium 5.8 percent, France 5.0 percent, Great Britain 3.1 percent, and Spain 3.8 percent.[5] Women are prescribed benzodiazepines at twice the rate of men, and the elderly are prescribed them more than those who are younger. The typical user tends to be an older woman with medical problems who is in substantial psychological distress.[6]

THE BENZO BLUES

I learned about these drugs and many other forms of talk therapy, behavioral techniques, and medications in my medical and psychiatric training. When I entered into practice, I saw that most forms of treatment helped the people who consulted me. Some patients improved through therapy alone. Some needed medications initially, then got better, went off the medications, and moved on.

I noticed, however, that patients with anxiety didn't seem to get better when I prescribed benzos month after month. I had always been concerned about prescribing these drugs for anxiety because I knew that they were habit-forming and had to be tapered slowly in order to avoid unpleasant, and even dangerous, withdrawal effects. The problem I kept having was that many patients were unable to get off benzodiazepines even when they wanted to.

I began to realize that people who took these drugs over the long term were plagued by anxiety and problems in their life *in spite* of all their treatment. Although they seemed to make some progress, they continued to rely on the drugs because their anxiety never resolved. I realized that each of the people who were stuck on benzodiazepines experienced the same set of problems, a specific behavioral syndrome that I call the Benzo Blues. The three major characteristics of the Benzo Blues are:

1. Ongoing anxiety
2. Physical or psychological dependence on benzodiazepines
3. Poor functioning in daily life.

Ongoing Anxiety

There are, in turn, three aspects to the experience of anxiety when someone is dependent on benzodiazepines. First *they continue to experience significant anxiety.* Although these drugs temporarily suppress the unpleasant physical and psychological *sensations* of anxiety, they do nothing to change the *process* of anxiety.

Some clinicians call anxiety a disease in order to emphasize that it is not just a random collection of unpleasant sensations but a unique, ongoing process with characteristic symptoms, time course, and associated problems that require specific treatment. The difference between the sensations and the process of anxiety is like the difference between the abdominal pain of an ulcer and the ulcer itself. The pain of an ulcer is unpleasant and leads sufferers to seek some form of relief. The correct treatment for an ulcer isn't a narcotic to relieve the pain, however, but medicine, or even surgery, that aims to reverse the disease process of the ulcer itself. This difference is crucial in understanding why anxious people who take benzodiazepines don't improve, even though they feel "better." The drugs can dull the "pain" of anxiety—but the process itself goes on.

By taking away the "pain" of anxiety, benzodiazepines allow a person to avoid confronting and resolving the uncomfortable situation that is leading them to be anxious. What should be a time-limited episode of acute anxiety can become transformed into an indefinite period of chronic anxiety.

The oscillation of the level of anxiety as the drugs take effect and then wear off leads to the second aspect of the experience of anxiety: *People are unable to manage their anxiety and become its victim.* These victims feel that they will not overcome their anxiety and must live with it as a constant presence in their life. Anxiety is no longer an unpleasant experience happening *to* them. Instead, anxiety has become *part* of them. Each time they take a pill, they say to themselves, "I can't manage anxiety on my own because it's too much for me." Because this happens over and over, they develop the belief that anxiety will always overwhelm them. They make a fundamental decision about anxiety: They decide that they can't handle it. They resign themselves to a life of anxiety.

Even when one experiences it regularly, anxiety is extremely unpleasant. This leads people to attempt to minimize the intensity of the sensations of anxiety while still leading their lives. The third aspect of their anxiety experience, then, is that *they use anxiety as a compass* that leads them toward some activities and away from others. For example, Susan was fearful of having another panic attack and gave up thinking she could ever live a life free of anxiety. She spent her time trying to "control" her life—i.e., to avoid anxiety whenever possible. When anxiety threatened her in one direction, she went the other way, even if the anxiety had to do with something she actually wanted. She was no longer the director in her life but was herself controlled by anxiety. The intensity of anxiety became a compass that guided her life.

Dependence

Dependence on benzodiazepines can be physical or emotional and is usually both. Physical dependence occurs after approximately four weeks of regular use and is characterized by the return of the symptoms of anxiety when the dose wears off. Although there are some pharmacological differences in terms of how each particular drug is absorbed, metabolized, and excreted by the body, they are all essentially equivalent in their ability to produce dependency.

Psychological dependence begins when people develop the *expectation* that the medication will help them. This expectation intensifies; the longer the drugs are taken, the greater the reinforcement of the beliefs that strengthen psychological dependency. The first belief is that they can't manage anxiety on their own, and the second is that they can manage it with the drug. The patient begins to feel, "I can't get through this alone." A psychological dependency is most obvious when a person gets relief from anxiety within a few minutes of taking the pill, long before the thirty to sixty minutes necessary for absorption of the drug from the intestines and transport to the brain.

After months of benzodiazepines, some people cut down their use to an "as needed" basis. They may use them only once or twice a week. Sometimes they carry them at all times so that they will have the drug if they "need" one. Although they are not physically dependent on the drugs, they still are psychologically dependent. This can be enormously destructive to a person's sense of well-being even in the absence of a true physical dependency. Thus, a person can still experience the Benzo Blues even without using benzodiazepines daily.

When people think of themselves as having chronic anxiety, they have transitioned into chronic benzodiazepine use, in which they have no active plan to stop taking the drug. This transition generally takes some months of regular use. People with intense anxiety, like the panic attacks that Susan experienced, sometimes make the transition to chronic benzodiazepine use in a matter of weeks.

Poor Functioning in Daily Life

Using anxiety as a compass and benzodiazepines as their only aid, chronic users retreat from full participation in their lives. They may function in their jobs and maintain some relationships with others, but a zestful involvement in life is replaced with a constricted outlook and style. The goal of each day becomes minimizing anxiety, not enjoying pleasurable activities. New opportunities aren't pursued.

WHY BENZODIAZEPINES SHOULD NOT BE USED FOR CHRONIC ANXIETY

Although people with the Benzo Blues can differ greatly in terms of their life circumstances, they all experience a common difficulty: They become preoccupied and overwhelmed by their anxiety and no longer see themselves as capable people who can manage their lives successfully because they now rely on a medication that they think helps them. The truth, however, is that benzodiazepines do not help people with chronic anxiety but actually work against them in a number of ways besides those noted above.

First and most important, *benzodiazepines simply don't help chronic anxiety.* Although they suppress the unpleasant sensations of anxiety for a few hours, the symptoms quickly return when the dose wears off. The tranquilizing effect leads people to think that they are being treated when they are not. The illusion of treatment provides a false reassurance that things will improve. But if benzodiazepines really worked, the chronic anxiety would end.

Second, *benzodiazepines have a number of negative effects that worsen a person's condition.* Foremost among these is the development of physical dependence, which causes patients to reexperience their symptoms of anxiety when they taper or decrease their dose. Other side effects include impaired memory and other thought processes, depression, and poor muscle coordination.

Some indirect effects include higher rates of motor vehicle accidents and hip fractures. Finally, there have been several reports in recent years that some chronic benzodiazepine users have areas of their brain that are abnormally small.

Third, *the vast majority of people who take benzodiazepines for chronic anxiety do not engage in other forms of treatment that are more effective.* This occurs in part because the drugs minimize the day-to-day distress of anxiety so that a patient's motivation to seek further care is substantially lowered. Using our previous example, a patient might ignore abdominal pain from an ulcer if he used codeine that was lying around the house from a previous visit to the dentist. Although he might feel better that day, the ulcer would worsen because the codeine allowed him to put off seeking more appropriate treatment. In a similar manner, use of a benzodiazepine allows people to put off treatment that is perhaps more difficult, painful, and costly but that would ultimately be more effective.

Finally, *when patients do not obtain effective treatment for their basic anxiety, they do not resolve the issues that overwhelmed them and led to the anxiety in the first place.* They remain mired in the Benzo Blues, and their lives stagnate. This deprives them of the chance to engage in new challenges and robs them of the benefits of new achievements.

If you have been using benzodiazepines for more than a month, are you experiencing any of the difficulties we've discussed? Are you still preoccupied with anxiety? Is the anxiety so terrible that you avoid facing what causes it? Do you watch the clock, waiting until you can take your next pill? Do you sometimes take extra pills when you are feeling especially anxious? Do you avoid activities that make you anxious? Do you feel you are overwhelmed with the problems in your life?

If you answer yes to some of these questions, then it is very likely that you are experiencing the Benzo Blues. However, it may be hard for you to accept that this is, in fact, a problem. Almost everyone on these drugs is surprised to learn that one of the main difficulties in overcoming their anxiety is continued use of the prescribed drugs *for* anxiety. Over the years, patients have used many arguments in an attempt to convince me that they do not have problems with benzodiazepines, and that they should keep taking them—arguments that you may be making to yourself right now. These arguments cluster around five issues.

COMMON OBJECTIONS TO THE CONCEPT OF THE BENZO BLUES

"Benzos Work for Me."

There is no question that benzodiazepines minimize the sensations of anxiety. Unfortunately, these sensations return within hours when the dose wears off. This leads to the ingestion of another pill, which "works" again. People focus their efforts each day on minimizing the unpleasant sensations of anxiety. So although benzodiazepines are temporarily effective on a superficial level, the process of anxiety continues.

If you really feel that benzodiazepines are "working" for you, why are you still anxious? If they were truly effective, wouldn't the relief you obtain allow you to move on to solve some of the problems that are leading you to be anxious?

"I'm Not an Addict."

Benzodiazepines are habit-forming, and people can have symptoms of withdrawal if they stop taking them abruptly. Does this make anyone who takes them an "addict"?

Significant confusion exists in both the medical community and the public about the meaning of the term *addict*. Some people use it to mean someone who regularly takes drugs to get "high." Other people use it to describe a person who takes more and more of the drug over time. Still others think than an addict is someone who becomes physically dependent on a drug and experiences withdrawal symptoms if he goes off it.

People who use benzodiazepines feel that they aren't addicts for three main reasons. First, they started taking the drugs for the relief of the extremely unpleasant physical and psychological experience of anxiety, not with an addict's hope of a kick. Second, they are taking their drugs under a doctor's order. Third, they generally don't use more of the drug than their doctor prescribes.

These are important distinctions. It is reasonable to reject the use of the term *addict* if it is used to mean someone who is taking drugs for kicks or who continually escalates the dose to get the same effect. However, the narrow definition of an addict as someone who experiences a withdrawal symptom does, unfortunately, apply to the vast majority of people who take benzodiazepines regularly. It is unfortunate in part because many people are never told that benzodiazepines cause dependency and are therefore shocked when they find that it is so hard to get off them. Whether one accepts or rejects the term *addict,* however, there is no question that physical dependency on benzodiazepines exists and causes significant distress.

"I Don't Take My Pills Very Often."

Many people think there is no problem if they take a small dose or if they take the drug infrequently. This is simply untrue and ignores the powerful effect a psychological dependency can have on a person's sense of themselves and on their ability to manage anxiety and the challenges of life. The Benzo Blues can occur whether one is taking 2 milligrams of Xanax four times a day or a quarter of a milligram every other day. Differences in dose and frequency are determined primarily by an individual's sensitivity to drugs, the severity of the anxiety, and the specific drug itself. People who are elderly or have slight frames generally require a smaller dose than younger people or those who are heavier, and those with severe anxiety generally require a larger dose. Xanax tends to be taken more frequently than Klonopin because of the way that it is metabolized by the body. The essential point doesn't change, though. Whether one takes a small or large dose, the problem is still the same: The taker feels incapable of managing anxiety and must reach for a pill when the symptoms start.

"It's Anxiety That Has Caused My Problems, Not the Benzos."

Anxiety can overwhelm people, lead them to feel like victims, and cause significant problems in their lives even if they have never been on benzodiazepines. A natural question, then, is: Are the Benzo Blues the result of the drugs or of the anxiety itself?

Anxiety itself clearly causes distress, but the regular use of benzodiazepines makes things worse. If you already feel incapable of handling anxiety, each additional pill will give you further evidence of your vulnerability and increase your sense of inadequacy. This vicious circle leads you to think that anxiety is the cause of your difficulties, but it's the drugs that keep that circle going.

"But I Can't Give Them Up."

Whenever I hear people say this, I am struck by how hopeless they feel. This hopelessness is unwarranted. I have seen teenagers, eighty-year-olds, people with severe anxiety, people who have been hooked on other drugs, and people who never wanted to come off benzodiazepines successfully taper and stop taking these drugs. In fact, the hopelessness people feel about stopping benzodiazepines is actually a subtle and pernicious effect of the drug itself. It is the voice of the drug inside you talking, not an accurate reflection of your true capabilities.

My answer to this objection is quite simple: Yes, you can. My certainty on this score comes from years of clinical experience. Anxiety is not some strange disease that strikes without warning or cause. Quite the contrary, anxiety, and the disorders of anxiety, can be understood by professionals and lay people alike. Effective treatments for anxiety exist that are straightforward, reliable, and well within the mainstream of standard medical practice.

I have seen too much pain to continue believing in benzodiazepines anymore. Continued use of these drugs for chronic anxiety is not reasonable, in spite of their popularity. I have developed an approach that has helped many people crippled by these drugs to stop taking them, to master their anxiety, and to move ahead in their lives. You can be one of those people.

· 2 ·

ANXIETY DISORDERS AND THE DEVELOPMENT OF THE BENZO BLUES

No two people are exactly alike. Consequently, people experience different aspects of the constellation of thoughts, feelings, sensations, and behaviors that constitute pathological anxiety in different ways, at different times, and at different levels of severity. Mental health professionals class these characteristics into a variety of anxiety disorders, which are described in detail in the *Diagnostic and Statistical Manual-IV*.[1] The development of the Benzo Blues varies depending on the individual and the anxiety disorder. Let's look at how people with anxiety disorders develop the Benzo Blues in their own unique way.

PANIC DISORDER

People with panic disorder experience panic attacks, in which there is a sudden onset of intense fearfulness that can last anywhere from a few minutes to a few hours and is often accompanied by palpitations, shortness of breath, sweating, chest pain, feelings of light-headedness, and thoughts of impending death. Panic attacks occur in a variety of psychiatric disorders. When they occur as the sole symptom of anxiety the diagnosis of panic disorder is made. Panic disorder can last for many years, causing intense personal distress and marked impairment of functioning.[2] Five percent of women will experience panic disorder at some point in their lives. For men, the rate is two percent.[3]

Panic attacks are extremely unpleasant and very distressing to experience. When I first saw Susan, whom I described briefly in chapter 1, she reminded me of this in no uncertain terms: "I'd never experienced anything as intense, unpleasant, and as overwhelming before. I was afraid I was going to die." Susan had been experiencing panic attacks for about five years. The second of three children, she had functioned well until the age of twenty-four, even though there had been, in her words, some "rough patches" during her growing-up years, owing to the fact that her parents quarreled a good deal.

After graduating from high school, Susan began working in retail. In time, she was promoted to the level of assistant manager, which included supervising shift assignments for thirty-five employees a week. When she was twenty-two she moved into an apartment with two friends. She had been dating since early high school and had several relationships that lasted more than a year. Susan met Mark when she was twenty-three. She immediately felt attracted to him because it "seemed like he knew what he was doing." As they grew closer, she could see that at times he could be somewhat domineering. This tendency was worse when Mark drank, but he always apologized for his behavior later. Although Susan didn't like Mark's drinking, she accepted his explanation that it was part of "having fun with the guys."

Susan told me that one day when she and Mark were driving to a restaurant, she suddenly began to feel her heart pounding hard and felt that she couldn't breathe. "I insisted that we go to an emergency room because I was sure I was having a heart attack. When the doctor told me that I was having a panic attack I didn't believe him at first. But he gave me a shot of Ativan and I felt better within half an hour. He gave me a prescription for Ativan pills and told me to take a pill two or three times a day whenever I needed to. He also told me I should go see a psychiatrist.

"Well, I had never thought of myself as somebody who was ever going to need a psychiatrist, so at first I refused. But the ER doctor explained to me that the physical sensations were actually part of a mental problem. He told me that he had seen a lot of people come in for panic attacks and that I could definitely be helped by a psychiatrist. So I decided to go.

"When I went to the psychiatrist, he asked me about my life. I told him I was satisfied with it. I liked my job. I was enjoying my relationship with Mark. We later broke up, but at the time we were getting along pretty well.

"The psychiatrist also asked me about my family. I explained that my mother had been anxious and pretty much stayed around the house. The psychiatrist then told me I had a 'chemical imbalance.' I told him that the Ativan really helped me, and he kept prescribing it."

As soon as I heard Susan tell me that she had a "chemical imbalance," I knew that we had a lot of work ahead of us. Many patients and doctors believe that a chemical imbalance means that there is a physical or physiological problem that causes anxiety. Susan's belief that she had a "chemical imbalance" minimized the significant contribution made to her anxiety by her experiences in life and the coping style she developed to manage problems. I was apprehensive when I asked my next question because I already suspected what Susan was going to tell me.

"Did you learn anything from those sessions with the psychiatrist about anything from the past that may have contributed to your symptoms of panic attacks and anxiety?"

"Not much. Let me think. I wasn't sexually abused or anything, if that's what you're getting at. My parents were nice to me and they cared about me. They didn't get along very well with each other, though, and they got a divorce when I was in high school. But I was spending most of my time out of the house anyway by then. I mean, I didn't like the fighting or the divorce, but it didn't affect me day to day. My father just moved a couple of blocks over. He was still around. But what good is it to talk about that stuff? I haven't thought about that time in my life for years, and it doesn't really bother me at all anymore. I get along okay with my parents now. That certainly doesn't have anything to do with why I have panic attacks."

"Did you continue to meet with the psychiatrist for psychotherapy?" I asked.

"Well, he recommended that I continue to see him in weekly sessions. But I didn't really see the point of it. It was expensive, it took a lot of time, and it didn't seem to go anywhere. I stopped seeing him for therapy, but I saw him every couple of months when we talked about the medication."

I know that many reasons can prevent psychotherapy from being productive. Sometimes psychotherapy "doesn't work" because the patient doesn't want to open up about her problems. Sometimes it is because the therapist is not sufficiently attuned to what the real issues are and as a result misses what is going on. Sometimes it is just not a good "fit" in the sense that the patient doesn't feel particularly comfortable with the therapist and the therapist is not able to bridge the gap. And, of course, some people cannot afford therapy or are unwilling to pay for it.

I knew that her experience with this psychiatrist was a crucial point in Susan's treatment for anxiety. Although she said that she didn't want to work on her problems because she didn't seem to have any, she still wanted to take the antianxiety medication. A more astute therapist might have been able to help Susan question why, if she had no problems, she nevertheless needed antianxiety medication. Psychotherapy can be used to focus on the areas that both parties think *may* cause some anxiety. As the work progresses, this kind of focus can point to the issues and events that *do* cause anxiety. Such work generally requires that therapists have faith in their own abilities to sort out the complexity of their patient's anxiety in spite of the resistance put up by the patient.

Oftentimes, both psychiatrists and patients avoid this work. Psychotherapy is often vague and frustrating until it is possible to clarify and focus on the real issues. Susan's psychiatrist shortchanged her by giving up too soon and continuing to prescribe benzodiazepines. He said, in effect, that she was powerless both to sort out the causes of her anxiety and to manage the sensations it caused. Of course, this devastating message wasn't stated overtly. Both Susan and her doctor thought they were doing the right thing. In fact, however, their lack of persistence constituted the first step toward Susan's case of the Benzo Blues.

When I know that someone has been taking benzodiazepines for an extended time, I question them very closely about their experience with anxiety after the panic attacks started and the medication was prescribed. The questions sometimes surprise them; many people are unaware of the effects that anxiety has on them. Nevertheless, it is essential to find out if they have been using anxiety and benzodiazepines as their compass to guide them through life. Susan admitted that she continued to be anxious even while taking Ativan.

"The Ativan worked at first. But I could feel that there were times when I might have a panic attack even with the Ativan.

Sometimes I'd take two. I found I didn't like to go shopping alone. I never got in a plane and flew, that's for sure; I still can't do that. You've got to help me with that. When I needed to go shopping, I'd go with other people or I'd sometimes take an extra dose of the Ativan. But there were times when I wouldn't take the Ativan at all. If I was just hanging around the house and nothing was happening, sometimes I'd skip a dose without any problem."

Susan clearly used her anxiety and benzodiazepine use as a compass. She experienced "anticipatory" anxiety, which occurs when a person fears that another panic attack may happen. Many people with panic attacks experience anticipatory anxiety, which leads them to be constantly anxious and on guard about what they are about to do even when they are not having a panic attack. Susan used the intensity of the anticipatory anxiety as part of her assessment of how much anxiety different activities would bring, how much she could tolerate, and whether she could engage in the activity. She gauged how stressful an event was likely to be if she skipped her Ativan, took the usual dose, or took an extra dose. She began to order her life according to how much anxiety she could tolerate and how much medication she took. In short order, Susan became a victim of anxiety and benzodiazepines. She was living her life under the mistaken belief that any event or occasion that caused her anxiety should be avoided because it was so unpleasant. Each time she took a pill that belief was reinforced in three ways.

First, each dose strengthened her belief that her anxiety was excessive and unwarranted. In reality, anxiety is unpleasant, sometimes extremely unpleasant, but it should not be seen as excessive or unwarranted. Anxiety is a natural feeling, unpleasant perhaps, like pain, but a natural feeling nevertheless. It is a call to action, a message from the body that something needs to be done differently. Second, each time Susan took a pill she was saying to herself that she needed to avoid anxiety. But anxiety needs to be confronted directly, rather than avoided, if it is to be overcome. Third, taking benzodiazepines reinforced Susan's belief that she was unable to handle anxiety on her own. I knew that Susan could overcome her anxiety, however; she just needed some tools other than benzodiazepines. I knew that this would be a difficult challenge for her because she had spent some years developing a now hardened belief that her anxiety disorder was a "chemical imbalance" that came into being for no reason.

I asked whether she had ever tried to taper off the Ativan and get along without it.

"I tried a couple of times," Susan replied. "I knew I couldn't stop cold turkey because I might go through some withdrawal. I know these drugs are addictive. I tried cutting my Ativan dose by taking it only once in the morning and at bedtime instead of three times a day. However, I found I just couldn't function without it. In the middle of the day I'd get real anxious. My psychiatrist told me that some people needed to take the medication three times a day and that there was no reason to take a lower dose if only the higher dose would help me."

"It sounds as if the anxiety was very unpleasant for you at that time," I said. "How were things going for you in general at that point?"

"Well, I stopped going to restaurants with Mark. I just felt so nervous there. It seemed like I couldn't calm down. I began having arguments with Mark about my anxiety and how it stopped me from doing things. Sometimes he was sympathetic, but sometimes he wasn't. We stopped getting along at all and finally broke up. I stayed at home mostly after that, which is how I got to be so comfortable with computers and landed this job. But over the last several years I've continued to have panic attacks once or twice a week, and I still dread them. I've been to a couple of therapists and another psychiatrist, but nothing has helped.

"I moved in with Kevin, my new boyfriend, about eighteen months ago. We've talked about marriage, but I want to hold off because I don't feel ready. Kevin is getting irritated with me, my anxiety, and my indecision. Periodically he gets angry and says that I should get off the pills. But then he apologizes. I have tried to get off a couple of times, mostly because he wanted me to. But every time I've tried I found that the anxiety about having another panic attack returned, so I stayed on the Ativan.

"I can't decide what to do about our relationship. I feel like I should get married, and I know that I love Kevin, but somehow the thought of getting married gets me even more anxious than usual. And now this new job is being offered to me, but I'm too scared to take it. I don't really know what to do. I feel like I can't move forward in my life. I'm stuck."

In fact, Susan *was* stuck. I knew that panic attacks and her fear that she would continue to experience panic attacks contributed to her inability to move forward. And I knew that benzodiazepines were contributing to her problems as well. I was also concerned because Susan clearly had no idea about what led her to have panic attacks in the first place.

I knew that treating Susan's anxiety would be difficult and improving the situation would require a significant commitment on her part. Some people who have accomplished this task have described it as the hardest thing they have ever done in their lives. They have also described it as the most worthwhile.

It is generally at this point that I begin to educate patients about the nature of anxiety and their drug use, and attempt to get them to share my hope that they can learn to master their anxiety, give up their benzodiazepines, and move forward in their lives. I generally start by exploring some of the reasons why they might be anxious, even though I don't know at the beginning exactly what they are.

"You've clearly had a very difficult time over the last couple of years with anxiety, Susan. Although the panic attacks seem to come out of nowhere, you say you are somewhat uneasy right now about making a commitment to Kevin to get married. Is it possible that some of the questions that you have about your present relationship were also troubling you about your relationship with Mark when the panic attacks started?"

"I don't know. It's kind of hard to remember back that far. I don't really think so, though. I suppose you always wonder whether or not you'll marry the person that you're with, but Mark and I never sat down and talked about it. We weren't really thinking of getting married then, so I wasn't even thinking about that kind of thing. I'm thinking about marriage now, though, in my relationship with Kevin. It's hard to make the commitment to marry Kevin. So many people are getting divorced these days you'd be a fool if you didn't think seriously about who you're marrying. Having your parents divorce isn't like dying or anything, but it just seemed like things were never the same after my parents split up for good. We did okay—I mean, financially things went okay—but I had the feeling that I never knew what was going to happen. My parents had separated before, and even though they always got back together, I never knew when things would fall apart again. When they split up for good, I felt helpless and that I couldn't depend on life turning out okay. I felt like I could rely only on myself. I suppose that's why I don't like to be in situations in which I'm unsure what's going to happen. I'm the kind of person who needs to be in control all the time. I don't like it when things surprise me."

As we talked about her preoccupation with maintaining control, Susan gradually acknowledged that she had fluttered on the edge of anxiety for many years during her childhood and after her parents' divorce because of their fighting and separations. She had been fearful of becoming involved with Mark because she didn't know how deeply she wanted to be involved with him when she didn't know what might happen in the relationship. She was able to tolerate her anxiety until the relationship with Mark deepened, and her anxiety about the stability of relationships increased beyond the point where she was able to contain it. At that point, the feelings of anxiety that she had long suppressed finally burst out of her.

It is unusual to be able to pinpoint with certainty all of a person's sources of anxiety in the first session; this generally requires more ongoing work in psychotherapy. Nevertheless, when a person is able to make some tentative connections, it bodes well for their capacity to master their anxiety in the future. Her acknowledgment that she had been experiencing some emotional turmoil prior to the onset of her anxiety made me feel hopeful that Susan wanted to learn how to master her anxiety, and not just try to suppress it with medication.

"It can definitely be done, though it can be difficult," I told her. "But the question is really more one of motivation. If you are willing to try, there is no reason that you cannot learn to manage your anxiety successfully and resolve some of your feelings about the issues that are contributing to it."

"We need to start by helping me get on a plane," Susan said.

"Before we talk about what is going to be helpful for you, we need to talk about your use of benzos. You've stated a number of times that you found it very helpful for you. Yet somehow here you are—still anxious, still having panic attacks, unable to accept a promotion, still unsure of your relationship with Kevin, and still unclear how to move forward in your life. I've seen a number of people who have taken benzos for extended periods of time, and they end up feeling as stuck in their lives as you are in yours. I've come to the realization that the drugs themselves contribute to being stuck, and I think this is the case with you.

"One of the ways that benzos contribute is that each time you take a pill you are saying to yourself that you can't manage anxiety on your own. In fact, however, there are very good ways you can learn to manage anxiety on your own without the help of medication. Secondly, there are other medications that can help you with panic attacks that do not have the negative effects benzos do." I looked closely at Susan to see her response. Sometimes people absolutely refuse to consider giving up their medication and I can never move them beyond the helplessness of the Benzo Blues to address the sources of their anxiety. No matter how reluctant people are to taper their medication, however, if they are willing to do it I know that they can get better.

"I don't think I could give them up right now," Susan said, "but I don't like staying on them. I know they're addictive. I'd like to try if you can help me do it."

"It's important that we go very slowly so that we don't cause you more anxiety than you are already experiencing. There are a number of medications that could be helpful for you at the beginning. But the main part of your treatment lies elsewhere," I said.

Susan had begun to see that anxiety was holding her back and that if she wanted to get better, she needed to do something different. What proved to be the most helpful for her was her willingness to look at issues in her life that could be contributing to her anxiety. Like many people with panic attacks, she responded well to a comprehensive approach that worked directly on both her symptoms and on the underlying causes for those symptoms.

PHOBIAS

Specific Phobia

Susan was very fearful of planes, to the point where she was even unable to get on a plane. Psychiatrists call such an intense and unreasonable fear of certain objects or situations a *phobia*. People can have phobias to almost anything in life. *DSM-IV* specifies four types of specific phobias: animals or insects; environmental situations such as storms, height, or water; receiving an injection or seeing blood; and situational, such as tunnels, flying, or driving.

Sometimes a phobia coexists with another anxiety disorder, as was the case for Susan, but frequently it appears alone.

I have never seen a patient with a circumscribed specific phobia become dependent on benzodiazepines unless there is another anxiety disorder such as panic attacks present. This is true in part because people troubled by a specific phobia are rarely limited by that phobia in other parts of their lives; most simply avoid the feared object or situation, and the inconvenience is relatively minor. A single dose of a drug can help the person participate in the event if it is absolutely necessary. In addition, behavioral treatments that are very effective without being particularly difficult are readily available for specific phobia.

Agoraphobia

As we have seen, in addition to her panic attacks and fear of flying, Susan was also somewhat fearful of restaurants and malls initially, although this faded with time. Sometimes, however, people with pathological anxiety stay at home as much as they can in order to avoid being in situations that might cause them to be anxious. The fearfulness that leads people to restrict themselves from open areas, crowds, or stores is called agoraphobia (literally "fear of the marketplace"). Seven percent of women will experience agoraphobia at some point in their lives, twice as many as men.[4]

Some people experience agoraphobia without ever having a panic attack, even though they may have had some symptoms of avoidance prior to the onset of agoraphobia.[5] One such person was Debbie, who was referred to me by her medical doctor.

"I have someone here that I'd like you to see. She's a twenty-three-year-old woman whom I first saw a couple of years ago when she had an abnormal Pap smear. When we first found the abnormality, Debbie was quite anxious, and I gave her a prescription for Librium. The cervical abnormality cleared up by itself over four months, but Debbie was very nervous during this time and kept taking Librium. She called the office for refills. Even after a good report on the follow-up Pap smear, she continued to be anxious about other things in her life and called for refills on the Librium. I last saw her about six months ago, and I told her then that I didn't think she should be taking the Librium any longer, but she assured me that it was still very helpful for her. She came in to see me today accompanied by her younger sister, who drove her. Apparently Debbie hasn't left the house for more than two months. She came in to see me today only because she's quite ill with fever and what appears to be pneumonia. I'll give her antibiotics for that, and I expect it will clear up without any difficulty. What I am most concerned about is that she hasn't been leaving the house, and she only came in today because her family insisted. She needs help."

We set up an appointment over the phone for me to see Debbie. I wondered whether or not she would be able to keep the appointment because of her obvious fear of going outside. I called Debbie at home and discussed briefly what the referring physician had told me and reassured her that I very much wanted to help. I knew a strong bond would be important if we were to get her out of the hole that she found herself in. I urged her to come for the appointment, and she agreed she would. In fact, however, she did not show up for her first appointment. When I called, she acknowledged that she was too afraid to leave the house. Her mother had been planning to take her but was delayed in getting home, and Debbie didn't feel that she could get to my office alone. We rescheduled for later in the week. Her mother brought her to our second appointment and stayed in the waiting room until we finished.

"I'm sorry I missed the first appointment," were Debbie's first words.

"I've heard how difficult it is for you to leave your house from your doctor and from you when we spoke on the phone. I know how hard that can be sometimes for people. I can understand that coming alone was not something you felt able to do earlier in the week, but I am glad to see you today. Tell me how things got to such a state in your life, and how you hope I can be of help."

"Well, I've always been on the shy side. I had a few friends when I was a little kid, but no one very close. I didn't like to have kids come over to my house because my father would make fun of them. He used to drink a lot and he would sometimes get mean. My mother would drink, too, though she wouldn't get mean; she would just stop paying attention to anyone around her. They are both better since they've stopped drinking a few years ago.

"When I was in second grade, I didn't want to go to school, and my parents really had to make me. They took me to the school psychologist at the time, who said that there really wasn't anything to do except force me to go to school. My parents used to drive me to school and then pick me up afterward. I went, but I never really felt comfortable being around so many people. I hated raising my hand in class even though I'm pretty smart. I never wanted to get up in front of the class and give a report or make a presentation. Making an oral presentation was one of the requirements in sophomore year in high school, and I just didn't do it. I actually failed that portion of my English class rather than go through with it. My parents never found out.

"But it wasn't like I never got out. I saw friends and did some dating. There was never anything too serious with boys, but it wasn't like I was a shut-in or anything. I finished high school and went to work for an accountant as a secretary. It was a quiet office and he was very nice. After I had been there a couple of years he even gave me health insurance benefits. He said that he would help me get an associate's degree in accounting and that my pay would rise because of that. I didn't really take him up on that because right after that I had the abnormal Pap smear."

"That can be a pretty scary thing for anybody," I said. "What was it like for you?"

"I was scared to death. I'd always worried that somebody close to me was going to die of an illness, but here it was me who was sick. Dr. Loomis was really nice to me, though. She tried to reassure me that the abnormality was a very mild one. She said that many people got better on their own without any treatment and that all we needed to do was follow up with another Pap smear in four months and see what it looked like at that time. I was upset, though, and she could obviously see it. She asked me if I wanted a prescription for Librium to help me calm down, and I said yes. I figured I probably wouldn't use it, but if I needed it, I'd have it."

"How were those four months for you waiting for the retest?"

"Terrible. I had difficulty sleeping at times. It was hard for me to concentrate at work, although I was able to do everything I needed to. I didn't really want to do anything else and mostly just went to work and came home. Some of my friends came by sometimes and were supportive, but I just really didn't want to leave the house."

"Did you use the Librium?"

"I used it to sleep off and on. And in the beginning I used it during the day as well. As the weeks went on, I used it less and less.

But as I got closer to the recheck, I got more and more anxious about the results, and I began using the Librium every day just to calm me down so I could actually get out of the house and get to work.

"The weird thing was that when Dr. Loomis told me that my test was normal, I was still anxious. I was glad that the test was normal and left her office that day thinking things were going to be fine. But the next day when I woke up I still felt worried about leaving the house. I didn't seem to have too much of a problem going to work at first, but I still didn't want to do anything else. Friends would call, but I just felt too uncomfortable to go out. I hated going shopping because I didn't like being in a crowd. Luckily, I live with my parents, and so either my mother would do the shopping or I would wait until I could go with her. I even did my banking at those twenty-four-hour machines so I wouldn't have to wait in line or talk to anybody. I haven't gone over the bridges out of town since that time. I just get too nervous every time I even think about them."

"Did you ever have a period of intense anxiety where you felt anxious, and were perhaps short of breath, with heart palpitations and feelings of dizziness?" I wanted to find out if she had panic attacks, since most people with agoraphobia do.

"I've never actually had an anxiety attack," Debbie said, "but I have been really worried that I might have one a lot of times. The times when I would have to go out, I would generally take the Librium, and that seemed to help calm me down a little bit. I don't really like being dependent on a medication. But it's the only thing that helps."

"When I spoke with Dr. Loomis on the phone, she told me that you hadn't left your house in two months. Have you stopped working?"

"I hung in there at my job as long as I could. But about three months ago I just could not get myself to go out anymore. I'd been taking Librium in order to get to work. I even used to take another one at work just to make it through the afternoon, but as soon as I could feel it wear off I would have to get out of there. I felt like it was torture to go to work. It wasn't like my boss was mean to me or anything; He was very nice and supportive. I know it's just me torturing myself somehow."

"Did you ever consider seeing a therapist or a psychiatrist before?"

"Well, my mother kept telling me I should see a therapist. But I didn't really know anybody, and I didn't want to leave the house to see anybody. I'm really only here because I've known Dr. Loomis for many years and she spent a lot of time telling me that there were treatments for what I've got. She said the term to describe it is agoraphobia, is that right?"

"The fearfulness that you have about being outside in an open place is usually called agoraphobia," I said. "What do you know about it?"

"Well, I don't know very much about it at all except for what Dr. Loomis told me," Debbie said. "I just don't know how you're going to be able to help me. I'm already taking medication, and that doesn't seem to help me enough. My grandmother had this same kind of problem, too, so I guess it runs in the family. She never left the house. We used to make fun of her when I was growing up; we called her 'the ghost.' If it's genetic, I don't see what any psychiatrist can do."

Debbie was right about the genetic component to her anxiety. There are families whose members clearly experience more anxiety and have a much higher frequency of anxiety disorders than the average population. Sometimes one can even observe excessive shyness and fearfulness in the children in the first year or two of life. However, Debbie was wrong in her belief that agoraphobia is untreatable, although the work can be challenging for both patient and therapist alike.

Her hopelessness about her anxiety, which stemmed in part from years of hearing about what a lost cause her grandmother was, contributed to Debbie's acceptance of the situation. Dr. Loomis had unwittingly contributed to this by giving Debbie a partial treatment for her anxiety. Although the Librium definitely helped her during the period of time when she was worried about having cervical cancer, it actually made things worse in the long run. Although Debbie used the Librium on a fairly minimal basis, it was enough to keep her situation in equilibrium. This equilibrium, however, deprived her of the opportunity to get appropriate treatment for her anxiety when she first began experiencing it two years before. I think Dr. Loomis was aware that a referral should have been made long before her anxiety had worsened to the point of disabling agoraphobia. Whereas Susan had begun to develop the Benzo Blues within days of her first panic attack, Debbie had gradually drifted into it over many months.

I knew that Debbie's treatment would be complex if her condition was going to improve. She needed to educate herself about anxiety and agoraphobia. She needed to learn some practical skills for managing her anxiety through the use of relaxation techniques. She needed to gradually expose herself more and more to anxiety-provoking situations in the real world until she began to be able to lead her life again. And she needed to come off the benzodiazepines. People with agoraphobia can generally regain their former lives if they engage in such treatment.

Social Phobia

People with social phobia have a marked and persistent fear of social situations in which they might become embarrassed. These situations may include public addresses, eating, drinking, or using a rest room in public. People with social phobia invariably experience physical sensations of anxiety such as hand tremors, palpitations, sweating, diarrhea, or blushing when they are in the feared situation. They may even experience panic attacks, but they only occur in the triggering situation itself. *DSM-IV* states that anywhere from three to twenty percent of the population has some degree of social phobia, depending on the threshold used to determine distress. Fifteen percent of women will experience social phobia at some point in their lives, while for men the rate is eleven percent.[6]

When he came to see me, Tom, a twenty-eight-year-old bank loan officer, acknowledged that he had always been somewhat nervous in social situations. His company had switched health plans, and he wanted a refill of Tranxene. He had been taking it for about two years.

"It may seem kind of odd for someone as uncomfortable with meeting new people as I am to be in a customer service position, but the money is pretty good, and as long as I take the Tranxene there isn't too much of a problem," he told me.

"Have you always been uncomfortable with new people?" I asked.

"It's not so much that I'm uncomfortable with new people in general," he said. "It's really only when I am expected to perform in front of people and might embarrass myself, like making a presentation to a group at the bank. I'm fine if I meet people when I go out to the movies or a restaurant. I can fly in a plane with hundreds of people I don't know. But if I'm supposed to speak to a group or if I have to confront someone, I become really anxious. My throat dries up, my heart starts to pound, I begin to sweat, and I usually need to get to a bathroom."

Tom went on to relate that he had felt this way most of his life. His father was in the military, and his family had traveled around the country to different bases every few years. His father was very gregarious and teased him about his difficulty meeting new people. At times his father would ridicule him in front of strangers and introduce him as "my son, the social hermit." This obviously embarrassed Tom further. One time his father threw him into the pool in front of the rest of his swimming class to force him to learn to swim. His father would say at times like these that he was just trying to "toughen" Tom up, but it had the opposite effect—Tom tended to become more easily embarrassed. He didn't like getting up in front of the class when he was in school, and he disliked showering in the locker room after gym. He was fearful of approaching girls and didn't start dating until he was in college.

Tom majored in chemistry in college and hoped to go to graduate school, but when he didn't get accepted to a program right away, he took a job as a teller in a bank instead. He continued to experience anxiety that interfered with his enjoyment of life. He had already made several efforts to improve his ability to handle anxiety. As a teenager he had practiced meditation and exercised regularly. For a while he went to a psychologist who used biofeedback machines. He stopped meditation and relaxation practice after he started at the bank because he no longer had the time.

After three years at the bank, Tom got a new boss who was very intrusive and overbearing. Whereas his first boss had been friendly and relaxed, letting the tellers do their work without much supervision, his new boss was always pacing behind the tellers and watching them. Tom felt as if she was always trying to catch them stealing. Her overbearing manner reminded him of his father, which caused even more anxiety. When he saw his internist for a routine physical, he asked for something to help him stay calm and received a prescription for Tranxene. He would take a dose in the morning and feel well enough during the day to function without major difficulty.

This unsatisfying situation lasted for many months. Finally, Tom applied for an open position as loan officer and was accepted. Almost as soon as he got the job, however, he began to feel even more stress. He had anticipated that he would be processing loan applications and that most people whom he worked with would be relatively friendly. However, because of a change in the real estate market, his job soon developed into cleaning up troubled loans by squeezing those who could pay and foreclosing on those who could not. His new boss was sympathetic to his difficulties but expected him to accomplish the task.

"All of a sudden I found myself in the position of dreading my encounters with customers and any dealings I had with my boss. I felt like I was between a rock and a hard place. I felt anxious all the time. I had difficulty doing the job and received a poor performance evaluation from my boss. The Tranxene really helped me. I would take two in the morning and maybe another at noon if I had a meeting with the management of the bank. Sometimes I take it for sleep, though, if I know I've got a really tough day ahead of me. And I took a dose yesterday because my sister found a lump in her breast and had a biopsy. It turns out she's fine, luckily."

Tom went on to relate that his relationship with his girlfriend wasn't very satisfying to him. They had broken up a couple of times but gotten back together because neither of them had anyone else and neither wanted to be alone. Although they enjoyed each other's company, they rarely had sexual relations.

"I just don't know how to break it off with Mandy, or if I even want to. I don't have any other friends, really, except a couple of people at the bank that I occasionally see. I'd have to start dating again, and that's always been really difficult for me. I've always dreaded approaching someone new, and I hate the pressure of initiating a sexual relationship."

Tom was someone who had been experiencing anxiety for much of his life. Although he'd been able to cope with it to some degree for many years, the stress at his job led him to start taking Tranxene. Unfortunately, the stress only increased, and he used no other coping mechanisms, even those that had been helpful in the past to him. This led him to increase his dosage of Tranxene, but of course, this did nothing to change the stresses in his life. He found that he avoided making any new changes in his life, such as breaking off a relationship that was unsatisfying, because he didn't want to add to his discomfort.

The vast majority of people with social phobia function to some degree but can obtain significant improvement with some behavioral treatment directed at helping them overcome the intensity of their fears.

POSTTRAUMATIC STRESS DISORDER

Posttraumatic stress disorder (PTSD) is a psychiatric condition that has been recognized since the early part of the century and has received a great deal of public attention in the last twenty years. PTSD occurs in people who were confronted with an event that involved actual or threatened death or serious physical injury to themselves or others. These events include things such as combat in war, rape and sexual abuse, natural disasters such as hurricanes or earthquakes, and car accidents. Following the traumatic event, a person with PTSD continues to vividly recall aspects of the event, generally avoids anything that might remind him of the trauma, experiences a general numbing of feelings, and has symptoms of increased arousal such as difficulty falling asleep, difficulty concentrating, hypervigilance or the feeling of being constantly "on alert," and an exaggerated startle response. People who experience these symptoms for less than one month are given the diagnosis of acute stress disorder, to distinguish it from PTSD, which lasts at least a month and can go on for decades.

The general public first became aware of PTSD when soldiers returning from Vietnam experienced flashbacks and hallucinations and on rare occasions had experiences in which they imagined themselves back in combat again. Public awareness has been focused more recently on women who have been diagnosed with PTSD because they were sexually abused as children or raped as adults.

I got a call about Sam, a patient with PTSD, from a therapist who runs groups for veterans. The therapist told me that Sam had called him up for an evaluation for his group because he had recently moved to the area. The therapist was concerned because

Sam was taking benzodiazepines, and he wondered if other medication might not be more effective for him.

I was struck, as I often am when I first see people with PTSD, at Sam's level of energy from the moment that he walked into my office. I was surprised at his appearance, because he looked about fifteen years older than his actual age of forty-two. I told him that I was familiar with some of what he was experiencing because of information I had received from the therapist from the veterans' group, and that I wanted to know how I could be of help to him.

"Well, I don't know that you really can. James, the group leader, thought I should see you. I need somebody to fill my prescription for Valium, but I don't really need anything more than that."

"I understand that you have been on the medication for many years, and that James wondered whether or not other medications might be of help to you."

"I've been on all of them. They've given me Elavil, Tofranil, Stelazine, Mellaril, Xanax, lithium—you name it, I've taken it. The VA has been giving me drugs for years. Valium is the only thing that has ever really helped."

"What symptoms do you have that are so troubling to you?" I asked. I could see that Sam was somewhat antagonistic, but if I was going to help him I needed to learn something about his current symptoms, what his past symptoms had been, and what his combat experience was, so that we could both be realistic about what I could do for him.

"I've had 'em all—the nightmares, the dreams, the rage attacks, anxiety, depression. The memories just don't go away."

"What was your experience in Vietnam?"

"I was never shot at myself. But I saw people coming back who had been shot. I lost a couple of friends there. One stepped on a mine. One never came back from patrol. We all went out looking for him the next day but we couldn't find him at that time. I knew I could have been the one lost out there instead of him.

"I was young going in—I was only eighteen. I thought I could handle anything when I was on my way over. But it was more intense than anything I'd imagined. It overwhelmed me. And the way we were treated when we came back made it worse. We got absolutely no support, and a lot of people hated us like the war was our fault. It's gotten a little bit better over the years since people realized that we were just doing a job—and we were trying to do a good job—that we weren't evil. But at the time the only place you got any kind of support from anybody was from other veterans and at the VA. That was the only thing that was good about the VA: People didn't think you were crazy. They didn't understand what to do for you, though."

"Did anything help?"

"Not really. I used a lot of drugs early on, like marijuana and alcohol. The drug use really caused me problems in my life. Part of the problem was me and the way that I acted, but the drugs really seemed to make it worse. I gradually stopped all the drug use with the help of AA and the Valium, really. I think without the Valium I might end up using street drugs again."

"How did the war affect your ability to develop personal relationships?"

"I could barely even talk to people for a couple of years after I got out. Friends I had from before I went overseas didn't really understand me, and I found it hard to relate to their concerns. I'd have brief relationships with girls, but my life was so chaotic that I never got anywhere with them. After I stopped the drug use in my late twenties, it got a lot better. I got my Realtor's license and I've been supporting myself that way for the last twelve years. I've been married and divorced twice. The first one was lucky to last a couple of years; it was in my twenties, when I was doing the drugs. I was married again in my thirties, but my wife was always complaining because I never really wanted to talk very much. I didn't really want to have kids because I'm not sure I could ever handle the crying. It's all I can do to handle myself. We finally split up about a year or so ago, and the divorce just became final about six months ago. She just got tired of me being so intense and wired up—and I can't really blame her."

"I know that you're in James's group, and he told me that you've been in other groups before. Have you ever seen a therapist individually before?"

"I saw one when I was doing all those drugs. It never went anywhere and it wasn't helpful at all. He kept wanting me to talk about the war and I didn't really want to talk about it, although it was hard for me to think about anything else. I feel much more comfortable in groups where other people have gone through what I have and I don't feel like I have to explain myself."

"Groups can be very effective for just the reason you are describing," I said. "Most people can feel significant emotional support from sharing their experiences with other people who have gone through what you have. But most groups that focus on issues like the war do not do any kind of detailed work in learning to manage anxiety effectively without drugs. Were you ever involved in a group or individual treatment that focused specifically on learning to manage your symptoms of anxiety?"

"People have tried to teach me relaxation techniques. They don't work for me. I've tried them a couple of times and they don't do anything for me."

"Did you ever practice them regularly?" I asked, knowing that only with sustained practice of relaxation techniques do people derive any benefit.

"No. The only thing that really works is the Valium. I take it once or twice a day and bedtime. There is sort of a hangover in the morning and I feel a little tired, but a couple cups of coffee and I'm right back up there. Real estate is the kind of business where you've got to hustle all the time."

"How much coffee would you say you drink?"

"Probably eight to ten cups over the course of the day."

"Do you notice that the coffee makes you more anxious?"

"Well, it gets me going in the morning and helps me keep my edge during the day. I never really noticed that it made me more anxious. I just know that I start to get tired toward the end of the day without the coffee. I know what you're getting at, though. You think maybe I use the coffee to wake me up from the Valium, and I use the Valium to calm me down from the coffee. I suppose there's a little bit of truth to that. But I know that I can't get along without the Valium. I've tried a couple of times and my anxiety just skyrockets. One time I started picking up drinking again."

Many people use caffeine while they're using benzodiazepines. The drugs cause a mental slowing, and the caffeine brings their thinking back to its usual speed. Unfortunately, although it improves their thinking, caffeine significantly increases their anxiety. Caffeine alone does not cause anxiety or benzodiazepine dependence, but it can exacerbate both conditions.

I liked Sam immediately because of his forthright manner, which even bordered on belligerence at times. I was concerned that he might be so angry at his previous experiences with treatment that he wouldn't be willing to consider a somewhat different approach. On the other hand, the therapy he had tried was not aimed at helping both his anxiety and his drug use. I know that people with PTSD can get significant relief from their day-to-day symptoms of hyperarousal with proper treatment, even if they continue to experience emotional distress about the trauma itself. When I began to detail this treatment, Sam was skeptical because of the lack of success that he had experienced with other forms of therapy in the past. He said he was willing to try, however, noting that "it couldn't be worse than what I've already been through."

Another patient, who I will call Betsy, developed PTSD and the Benzo Blues not from an extended traumatic experience over years, but from a single event.

Betsy was fifty-five years old when I first saw her. She had taught music at a junior high school for many years. She was cleaning up the music room one day after band practice when the janitor came in and began moving some of the furniture around. After he had finished mopping the floor and putting chairs back, he left the room. Neither of them realized that he had left his cigar behind. It had fallen onto the floor and rolled over to the wall, where it ignited papers at the bottom of the bulletin board. The flames grew extremely quickly. The fire extinguisher was on the wall by the bulletin board and couldn't be reached because it was surrounded by flames. Betsy was afraid of trying to get out the door because in order to do so she would have to go very close to the flames. There was a great deal of smoke; though the sprinkler system went on, the flames weren't immediately extinguished because the wall had caught fire. Betsy attempted to open one of the windows and escape through that, but the windows were painted shut. She finally threw a chair through the window and was able to make it out without any significant harm to herself. Because the smoke alarms had gone off fairly quickly and the fire department arrived promptly, there was only moderate damage to her room and none to the rest of the school. Nevertheless, Betsy had been extremely frightened. The fire department ambulance brought her down to the emergency room for evaluation. Although she had no significant medical problems, she was quite upset and tearful. The emergency room nurses called her husband, who came down immediately, but even he was unable to calm her down.

"I thought I was going to die," she told him. The emergency

room physician gave her a prescription for Klonopin. Over the next few days she continued to be quite tearful. She felt that her reaction to the fire was excessive, but she could not stop herself from feeling so upset. Betsy continued to use the Klonopin regularly over the next few weeks. She began having difficulty sleeping because of dreams about the fire. Sometimes the dreams were much more elaborate and dramatic than the actual fire had been, and she would awaken bathed in sweat.

She found it increasingly difficult to go back to school even though the fire damage had been repaired within a matter of days. She felt she was being unreasonable, but every time she went into the music room she became increasingly anxious. At times she would have panic attacks. She used the Klonopin to help calm her down, but it wasn't enough.

Betsy felt lucky that the fire had occurred in late May so that she could use the summer vacation to try to regroup. Over the summer, however, she continued to be somewhat anxious and stayed on the Klonopin. She kept hoping that with time the intensity of her anxiety would diminish. Unfortunately, she became increasingly anxious as September and the beginning of the school year approached. She spoke to the principal and asked to have the music classes moved to another classroom. The principal was able to help her move to another classroom because another teacher was sympathetic to Betsy's plight and wanted to help as much as possible. Although Betsy felt temporarily better for some days while she was preparing her new room, she was aware that her anxiety was continuing.

The first few days of school seemed to be fine. She had always enjoyed teaching, and during the day teaching took her mind off her worries. In the past she had stayed late to provide violin lessons for some of her students and to lead the band practice. Now, however, she found herself increasingly anxious about staying late and being one of the only adults in the building after classes were over for the day. She found another music teacher who could take over the band practice because she finally felt incapable of doing it herself. She just felt extremely anxious when she was the only adult in the building besides the janitor.

As the school year progressed, Betsy continued to have difficulty going to the school. She continued to have dreams about fires. She became upset and anxious if she saw stories about fires in the newspaper or on television. Although the Klonopin had seemed to help her for the first month or two, she regularly had nightmares involving fires and often did not get an adequate amount of sleep. She continued to be distraught throughout the school year. She was able to make it to work but found that she had lost any pleasure—in teaching and in the rest of her life—because of the fire and her reaction to it. She continued to take Klonopin, thinking it was helping her to function during the day.

I saw Betsy after she had finished that school year and was considering retiring. Her principal had recommended that she come in for evaluation. She had been an excellent teacher for many years, and they didn't want to lose her. She hoped that Betsy would be able to get some help.

I was struck by two aspects of Betsy's experience when we first met. First, although she had been able to function somewhat in spite of her PTSD, she had withdrawn from significant aspects of her life that had previously given her pleasure. She had given up leading band practice, which was the school activity that she had always enjoyed the most. She no longer taught students after school individually or in small groups, which had been another source of pleasure for her, and of additional income as well. That she was considering retiring early concerned me greatly. The other aspect of Betsy's experience that troubled me was that she had never received any adequate psychiatric treatment. Many people who have traumatic experiences as adults benefit enormously from treatment that helps them to address the feelings that arise from the trauma and the symptoms of physiological hyperarousal. Although people had recommended that Betsy see a counselor, she didn't really want to and kept hoping that she would be able to get better on her own. She kept getting the medication from her family physician, who had recommended counseling several times. However, Betsy never took the referral and her doctor kept prescribing the medication.

One of the subtle but pernicious problems with chronic benzodiazepine use is that people feel that the relief they get from the pills is good enough, so they do not seek additional treatment. Although this may seem reasonable, a problem arises in that they often don't work on resolving the root cause of their anxiety. Benzodiazepines actually interfere with such efforts at resolution because patients do not pursue a more intensive treatment. Sometimes they are fearful of what they will find. Sometimes it is too expensive. Sometimes they have misconceptions about what psychological treatment will involve or they may have a lifelong style of covering things up rather than trying to work on their emotional problems. Whatever the reason, people who use these drugs chronically generally have not engaged in sufficient additional treatment to help them get to the root of their anxiety, learn to master the symptoms of anxiety that they do experience, and move on in their lives.

GENERALIZED ANXIETY DISORDER

People with generalized anxiety disorder (GAD) experience excessive worry about many of the events and activities in their lives—to the point where it interferes with their ability to function. It is unusual to see a pure form of generalized anxiety disorder. Sometimes people also experience panic attacks or depression. Even when they do not experience panic attacks, however, they worry excessively about day-to-day matters. They may worry about possible misfortune to a child who is in no danger. They may worry that an abnormal physical sensation constitutes evidence of a life-threatening condition like cancer, even though this is unrealistic. They may worry about finances even when there is no cause for concern. GAD is experienced by 6.6 percent of women at some point in their lives; for men the rate of GAD is 3.6 percent.[7]

When I first met with Marilyn, the fifty-two-year-old woman whose husband had unexpectedly died of a heart attack three years before, it was unclear to me whether her problems were primarily due to GAD or whether she was depressed.

Marilyn told me that she had grown up in a small town with two older brothers. Her father worked as a laborer in a local mill, and her mother stayed home to take care of the children. Her parents had traditional roles in the marriage. Her father tended to make the financial decisions. Her father cared deeply about the children but was unable to spend much time with them because of the amount of work he did. However, he insisted that he be consulted for even minor household decisions, such as how much time the children had to spend on their homework, or which friends they could see. If he was not consulted, he became angry. Marilyn's mother deferred to him even if she thought he was wrong in order to "preserve the peace."

When Marilyn was thirteen her mother died of pneumonia. While this was obviously difficult for her and the rest of the family, this was the time when she "grew up." She already knew how to cook and now took on the role of shopping and preparing the meals at home. Her father continued to take an active role in the house, and like her mother before her, Marilyn would defer to him even on issues that she felt strongly about. For example, she wanted to go to college after high school. Her father, however, got her a job as a secretary in an insurance company and convinced her to take it because the money was stable and there were opportunities for advancement. He felt that there was no point in sending Marilyn to college because she would probably never use the education to advance herself after she had married and had children.

The decision to forgo college was deeply distressing to Marilyn. She was giving up not only a long-held wish, but one that she and her mother had talked about many times before her mother's untimely death. Her mother had always wanted to pursue nursing and had impressed upon Marilyn the importance of self-improvement and self-reliance. Marilyn missed her mother's presence terribly during those first few years, but never more than when her father refused to send her to college. She felt that if her mother had been there to lend her support and encouragement, she would have been able to convince her father to send her to school. Marilyn felt that after her mother died, she was unable to establish a satisfying balance between pursuing her own wishes and helping others. She took the job he recommended.

Marilyn met her husband on the job. He was four years her senior and a salesman. Her father approved of him, and they married soon after they met. She became pregnant quickly and quit her secretarial job to stay home with her children. Marilyn and her husband were comfortable financially and satisfied with their lives. Her husband tended to make the financial decisions, while she concentrated on her involvement with their children.

At the time of her husband's death, things had been going fairly well. The two older children had been to college and had started families of their own. The youngest child was still at home, finishing his final year of high school. As anybody would be, Marilyn was extremely distraught at her husband's death. She felt alone. Her husband was such an important part of her life that she didn't know how she would go on. With the support of her family, however, she got through the funeral without a major breakdown. But Marilyn began experiencing difficulties after the funeral was over. Her routine and the activities that had been so satisfying now seemed empty to her. She was often restless during the day and fatigued easily. She had difficulty concentrating. At times she felt anxious. She wasn't sure what specifically she was anxious about, but she knew that she missed her husband. She began having difficulty sleeping at night.

She also had brief periods when she would become short of breath and have palpitations, and she worried that she was having a heart attack. Marilyn then made an appointment with her physician, who pronounced her healthy. She mentioned her difficulty sleeping and was given a prescription for Dalmane. She was told to try to avoid using it every night so as not to become dependent on it. Over some weeks, however, she found that she was unable to sleep when she did not use the Dalmane and did begin using it every night.

Marilyn continued to be intermittently anxious during the day. As her husband's estate was sorted out, it became clear that although there was no immediate problem with Marilyn's finances, she would not have enough money to support herself. She and her husband had spent a great deal of their money in financing their children's college educations, and only a modest savings account remained. Although her husband had life insurance, some of it had to be used to pay the medical expenses surrounding his death. Most would be needed to pay for her youngest son's college tuition, which Marilyn was determined to pay for now that her husband was no longer bringing in a paycheck. Marilyn could see that the remaining amount would soon be inadequate because of the mortgage and car payments that she needed to make. Nevertheless, she did have enough to meet her expenses in the months following his death.

When Marilyn saw her physician several months after her husband had died, he was concerned that she still was having difficulty sleeping. He continued her prescription of Dalmane. Additionally, he gave her a prescription for Xanax to help her feel less anxious during the day. At first she took the Xanax only a couple of days a week. However, she became more anxious when her youngest son announced that he planned to summer in another state after he graduated from high school. She was worried that after he left she wouldn't be able to maintain the house. She told me that she began using the Xanax two or three times a day when he announced that he was going to leave. After he left she continued to use it daily, and she found that when she had to do something stressful, such as meeting with her attorney to resolve issues of her husband's estate or when significant anniversaries arrived, she needed extras.

Over the course of approximately a year Marilyn's anxiety continued. She felt Xanax continued to help her, but her children grew increasingly concerned because they felt she wasn't coping well. She went to church regularly but no longer took part in any of the related activities that she had enjoyed previously. She stopped baby-sitting for her grandchildren, complaining of lack of energy. She stated that she was tired in the morning, and although coffee perked her up, she still didn't feel she had the energy to do very much. She continued to mourn the loss of her husband and cried intermittently. When she saw her physician a year and a half after her husband's death, he felt that she was depressed. He referred her to a psychiatrist, who prescribed Prozac. She did feel somewhat less depressed and less tearful on the antidepressant. The psychiatrist recommended that Marilyn "get out more" and do things to become more active in her life. But the things that he recommended made her feel more anxious, and she found herself unable and unwilling to pursue them. She didn't really feel comfortable with this psychiatrist and stopped seeing him. She remained on all three medications, however, which were now prescribed by her family physician.

Marilyn decided to move in with her daughter, who lived in the same town. Being in her own house was often very painful for her because everything reminded her of her husband. It made sense financially to sell the house so that she wouldn't have to keep up the mortgage payments and would be able to use some of the money from the sale of the house. Finally, she wouldn't feel as alone because she would be living with her daughter and her family.

After moving in with her daughter, Marilyn gave up her car because she was afraid of having an accident, even though she had always been a good driver. When she came in to see me, she was quite anxious and was still using Xanax two or three times a day, as well as Dalmane for sleep. She stated that her anxiety and insomnia worsened each time she tried to cut back on the Xanax or the Dalmane. She also told me that she had recently made several visits to her internist. Her complaints included frequent urination, nausea, and feelings of fatigue. However, her doctor found no medical causes that were contributing to her symptoms.

After I had met with Marilyn a couple of times it was clear to me that although she had been depressed somewhat since the death of her husband, her major difficulty was with chronic anxiety. It wasn't her depression or lack of energy that was holding her back; it was a chronic sense of apprehension about what the future might hold for her. She worried about her finances, her health, her energy level, and a host of other concerns.

Once again benzodiazepines played a very unfortunate role in worsening the difficulties caused by anxiety. Because they had given her enough relief during the day she had never been willing to pursue effective treatment for her problems. One result of this was that she spent an extended period of time on the pills during which the situation got neither worse nor better. This "plateau" can last for many years. Additionally, she developed some physical complaints. This is not uncommon. Many people with anxiety have numerous physical complaints for which no medical cause can be found. In fact, billions of dollars are spent each year on medical tests to rule out medical problems for symptoms that are induced by anxiety. Finally, Marilyn became depressed. Although Prozac helped, her depression was a sign that things were getting worse for her and that she needed more than just medication.

People with GAD generally need extensive psychotherapy because they need a lot of time to work on their current concerns and worries while still reserving some time to address the emotional roots of their anxiety. Many people need to see a psychiatrist for one to three years to improve sufficiently so that their anxiety no longer interferes with their life.

OBSESSIVE-COMPULSIVE DISORDER

Obsessive-compulsive disorder (OCD) is an anxiety disorder in which a person experiences recurring thoughts that are intrusive and inappropriate and that cause marked anxiety and stress. Common examples include fear of contamination, fear that they will hit or harm their children or other loved ones, or that their partners are unfaithful to them. Many people with obsessions also experience compulsions, which are repetitive behaviors or mental acts that people perform in response to an obsession. Common examples include hand washing, counting rituals of such things as license plates or lines in the sidewalk, and repeatedly checking lights and stoves to insure that they are turned off. People with OCD fully recognize that their thoughts and behaviors are inappropriate and unreasonable but feel powerless to stop them.

In recent years it has become increasingly clear that OCD is largely a biological disorder. Some researchers believe that it may be related to a disorder of attention, i.e., the person is unable to pay appropriate attention to their environment but instead becomes preoccupied by trying to organize irrelevant details. Other clinicians feel that OCD may be related to disorders such as schizophrenia because of the disorganization of the thought processes, even though the person retains his ability to distinguish reality from fantasy. OCD can be severely distressing and disabling. Almost every known treatment has been tried for it. Brain surgery has been used in the past and is still occasionally employed in intractable cases. It is no wonder that some people turn to benzodiazepines in an attempt to gain some relief.

There was no mistaking the intense distress that Peter, a twenty-six-year-old engineer who had symptoms of OCD for more than six years, was experiencing when he first came in for treatment. He had first noticed the symptoms of OCD in college as he was nearing graduation. He began worrying that he might develop AIDS. He lived in a college dormitory, and he became increasingly concerned about living in an environment with so many other people. He began showering numerous times a day and washing his hands incessantly, thinking that might remove any possibility of being infected. Intellectually, he knew that he could not contract AIDS from casual contact, but he was unable to reassure himself. He began cleaning his room daily, keeping everything in a specific position in order to reassure himself that no one had entered his room without his knowledge.

After Peter finished college, he had great difficulty obtaining work because of his fears of contamination. At that point he first sought psychiatric help. It was first thought that his symptoms were psychotic in nature, and he was given Thorazine and Haldol. These medications provided no benefit, and Peter experienced a number of unpleasant side effects from them. He stopped taking them almost immediately and continued to be quite distressed. He washed his hands upward of thirty times a day and spent hours doing counting and checking rituals.

He was next given Ativan and began using it regularly. He used large doses, up to 10 milligrams a day. He stayed on the Ativan at varying dosages for the next several years. He was able to find work as an engineer but was unable to participate in any social activities. A year prior to my evaluation he was placed on clomipramine, a relatively new medication that helps many people with OCD. His compulsions lessened, but he continued to experience significant obsessional thinking and stayed on both Ativan and clomipramine. When I first saw Peter, he said that the Ativan seemed to help him feel less bothered by the obsessions, although it slowed his thinking down a little bit. At times his muscular coordination was not good. He wondered if this was due to the Ativan and whether it would impair his ability to drive.

Unfortunately for Peter, there is no treatment that significantly improves OCD. Medications can sometimes be of some benefit, but they rarely provide dramatic improvement. Most people with OCD continue to experience significant distress despite all treatment. Benzodiazepines appear to offer some symptomatic benefits, but they often worsen functioning somewhat. Peter actually wanted to get off the Ativan because he was concerned about his ability to drive safely, and he felt that it worsened his memory when he was trying to learn new tasks. In fact poor muscular coordination and worsening memory are just two of the side effects that people experience with this class of drugs. These side effects are often overlooked because of the drug's supposed benefits, but astute self-observers such as Peter can often discern and dislike these subtle effects.

ADJUSTMENT DISORDER WITH ANXIETY

When people experience an excessive degree of anxiety in apparent response to some identifiable stress, but without any other symptoms of anxiety such as panic attacks or obsessions, their condition is given the label of "adjustment disorder with anxiety." This is one of the more common reasons people experience anxiety and come for treatment. If the anxiety is short-lived and the person "adjusts" to the stress, there is little chance that benzodiazepines will be taken for any extended period of time, even if they are prescribed initially. If a person fails to adjust to the stress and stays on the medication, however, then other factors need to be more fully explored and addressed.

Many physicians routinely chalk up their patients' problems to the current stress and apply this label without undertaking a full evaluation. They assume that the patient will get over their anxiety without too much difficulty or any lasting effects. Because their problems appear obvious, these patients often do not receive a complete evaluation that would tease out other factors that contribute to the anxiety, and as a result they never truly "adjust" to the stress.

When Jim was referred by his medical doctor because his anxiety hadn't improved after two years, it was clear to me that such had also been the case with him. He had first become anxious when his wife became pregnant, and both he and his physician had thought that his apprehension was merely due to his concern about his new role as a father. Although he and his wife had been attempting to conceive for some years, once she finally got pregnant, Jim found he couldn't enjoy it. He worried that something would happen to the baby before it was even born. He worried whether his wife and the baby would make it through childbirth without any problems. He worried about his ability to support his family financially. His worries increased to the point that he had difficulty sleeping. He finally asked his doctor for something to sleep and was prescribed Klonopin, which did help him to sleep.

Unfortunately, the stress in Jim's life increased. As the pregnancy progressed he grew increasingly preoccupied with the fact that his wife would stop working after the delivery and he would be the sole breadwinner. Jim had never had anyone truly depend on him before, and although they had some savings, and his wife planned on returning to work after a year or so, he didn't know if he could handle the increased responsibility. He no longer felt that he could leave a job if he didn't like it. He began to feel hemmed in. His sleeplessness and anxiety increased, and he began to use the Klonopin every night.

Jim grew more anxious during the day at work as well. His concentration slipped. Normally a meticulous worker, he made uncharacteristic mistakes. He began to work through his lunch break so that he could double-check his work. He spent more time working to insure that he got the job done and grew more distant from the people at work, with whom he usually enjoyed spending leisure time.

He thought he would feel better after the baby was born, but he continued to feel anxious. He was worried about his finances, but what was most troubling was that he felt nervous around the baby. He found it difficult to enjoy just being with her. He didn't mind feeding or diapering her, but he found it difficult to soothe the baby when she cried for other reasons. He just didn't feel comfortable holding the baby and let his wife do most of the actual hugging, cooing, kissing, etc. He sometimes took the Klonopin during the day as well just to feel more relaxed around his new daughter.

Then his wife became pregnant a second time unexpectedly. With this news, Jim felt even more pressure and anxiety because his wife wouldn't be able to go back to work when they planned. It was at this point that Jim saw his internist and broke down in tears. He said that he didn't know if he'd be able to keep functioning and was scared that he wouldn't be able to support his family. His internist finally referred him to me.

Jim told me that he has sworn to himself that he would never let his family down as he had been let down by his own father, who had died in a motorcycle accident when Jim was eight. As Jim grew older, he became increasingly angry because he thought his father had been irresponsible to ride on a motorcycle when he had children. He vowed that he would always take care of his family, and now he was worried that he wouldn't be able to.

Like many of the people I've described, Jim felt that the Klonopin was the only thing standing between him and a nervous breakdown. Unfortunately, the Klonopin was one of the causes bringing him to this point. The partial relief of anxiety afforded by the Klonopin allowed him to avoid seeking more time-consuming, expensive, and intensive treatment, but it was this kind of treatment that could have averted this crisis.

"UNSPECIFIED" ANXIETY

Some people experience significant anxiety that does not fit any of the patterns previously described. *DSM-IV* terms this problem "anxiety disorder, not otherwise specified" (ADNOS). This label was included in *DSM-IV* in order to insure that a person with symptoms of anxiety without the associated characteristics of other anxiety disorders could be given a diagnosis that would recognize the significant distress that anxiety was causing. *DSM-IV* acknowledges that no diagnostic scheme is perfect because of the incomplete understanding of the mind and brain in health and sickness, and this catchall term is used when a person's symptoms don't fit a recognized category.

Because of this, ADNOS is sometimes used cavalierly and incorrectly. This was the case with Janet, the elderly patient I briefly described in chapter 1. She acknowledged that she had always been a nervous person, but she had no specific symptoms of anxiety until the last couple of years. However, she had been experiencing flare-ups of colitis since adolescence and other medical problems since then. Knowing that colitis can often be exacerbated by anxiety, I asked Dr. Crandal, her internist who referred her to me, how she handled stressful situations in her life.

"Janet calls the office a lot with concerns about her physical health. It seems as though her medical conditions get worse when she's having problems. She first developed colitis at menopause. She hasn't really talked about it, but I know that menopause hit her pretty hard because she had always wanted children. She never had it easy. Janet's mother had to go to work when Janet was eleven because of the Depression, and she was left raising her younger brothers and sisters. By the time they had all grown up it was the middle of World War II, and she spent those years caring for one of her brothers who was wounded. After the war she cared for a sister who came down with tuberculosis. She rarely went out on dates. It seemed as if she was too independent to settle down with anyone.

"She never really faced what a mistake it was to stay single. She compensated by being the aunt who was always available to babysit for all her nieces and nephews, and that's kept her busy, but I've known her and other members of her family for more than twenty-five years, and I know that she's never really been happy. She won't admit it, though, she's the leader of the stiff-upper-lip club.

"I sent Janet to you because she seems to be getting worse. She calls the office all the time with one problem or another—headaches, insomnia, abdominal pains, muscle aches, feelings of being faint. She's had every test known to man, and we can never find anything really wrong with her. She knows the whole office staff by name because she's been in here so much. I don't know what to do with her anymore. She's been anxious for years. She doesn't have panic attacks or generalized anxiety, I've just called it an unspecified anxiety disorder—that's why I've got her on the Serax. She's taken it on and off for years, but now she's on it two or three times a day. And she seems just as anxious. At least she seems to come in just as much, maybe even more. Maybe she's got an underlying depression. I thought of adding some Prozac, but she's already on Serax, Restoril, and Fiorinol, and it seemed like I was getting in over my head."

Dr. Crandal's honesty about Janet's frequent complaints and his own feelings of helplessness helped me to understand that she was the kind of person who had difficulty directly discussing her feelings about events in her life. Rather than assert her own needs and desires in relationships, she ignored them and spent her energy taking care of others' needs. When facing stressful issues in her life, she would experience physical sensations of anxiety, misinterpret them as actual medical problems, and seek her doctor's evaluation. Besides being reassured that she was, in fact, healthy, she also secondarily enjoyed the attention given to her by members of the medical profession. However, Janet never truly resolved the anxiety that she felt about the troubling situations in her life. As these situations built up over the years, her anxiety worsened.

This unhealthy pattern of seeking medical evaluation for symptoms resulting from anxiety is, unfortunately, all too common. Many elderly people are unused to expressing their feelings directly because they grew up during times when economic survival was the dominant concern. The Great Depression, World War II, and epidemics of infectious disease such as polio and influenza left little room for acknowledging feelings and meeting one's emotional needs. But these needs don't go away just because they are ignored, and it is not unusual for them to arise during evaluations for physical problems.

It is also common for medical doctors to overemphasize the medical evaluation of such complaints by ordering every possible test—because they can't be sure that the problem isn't physical. The doctor thinks he is doing everything he can to reassure her, and himself, that he's leaving no stone unturned in his efforts to help her. At the same time, however, he unconsciously devalues the patient's psychological distress by prescribing medication without referring her to a psychiatrist for a full evaluation of what is leading her to be anxious. With Janet, Dr. Crandal fell into a common trap. He prescribed benzodiazepines somewhat carelessly—for "anxiety"—without a complete evaluation.

Although Janet technically meets the criteria for ADNOS, a more accurate label is "somatization disorder," which refers to someone with frequent medical complaints that are not caused by a general medical condition. Millions of people have somatization disorder, and they account for a disproportionate share of all the medical care provided in the United States. People with somatization disorder often receive poorly conceived treatment from medical doctors because they are like square pegs trying to fit into round holes. Though their real problems are psychological, they complain of physical problems. Physicians like Dr. Crandal concentrate on the details of the medical problems, missing the fact that the true problem is psychological distress.

In cases like this, benzodiazepines can seem like a good solution to both parties. Dr. Crandal sees the anxiety and knows that Serax can quiet her down. And Janet feels calmer with the medication and also feels that her distress is legitimized by having a doctor give her medication. Unfortunately, benzodiazepines allow both parties to proceed as if something were being done to help Janet's distress, when a true solution to her problems lies elsewhere. A better solution would be to help her face the things in her life that she feels anxious and distressed about—a task made harder because of years of unneeded medical tests and misguided treatment that allowed her to continue to avoid uncomfortable feelings.

The term ADNOS is also used to describe someone's anxiety when they experience anxiety and other difficulties functioning in a variety of areas for all of their adult life and when the anxiety is merely part of what they are struggling to manage and tolerate. They sometimes experience significant depression as well and have generally developed a coping style that is maladaptive and causes them and others distress. The etiology of their anxiety, depression, and coping styles is often not entirely clear. People with this form of chronic anxiety can be a challenge because treatment generally needs to be directed toward more areas of a person's life than just relief of symptoms of anxiety.

It became apparent when I first met Heather that her symptoms of anxiety were not easily compartmentalized into any of the disorders previously described. She was a smart, pretty twenty-eight-year-old. She came in for evaluation shortly after moving to the area because, she said, "I've seen psychiatrists for years and will probably always need to see one." She stated that she had been anxious for some years and was currently taking Zoloft, one of the newer antidepressants, and Xanax.

She said growing up had been difficult for her. Her parents had divorced when she was four. She initially lived with her mother for the next ten years or so, spending weekends with her father. Her father began to molest her sexually when she was ten. Although he refrained from intercourse, he fondled her and insisted that she masturbate him. He swore her to secrecy by threatening never to see her again if she told her mother. The molestation stopped when she was fourteen after she confessed to a teacher what was happening. Although she still visited with her father, she always had other people around and never stayed at his house again.

Heather became sexually active with boyfriends at sixteen. Relationships were intense but didn't last long. She started drinking beer by the age of sixteen and by eighteen was drinking it regularly when she went off to college. She grew depressed at one point and overdosed on aspirin but didn't pursue any psychiatric treatment. In college she smoked marijuana. Heather said that her drug use interfered with her attaining great success in college, but she was able to go to law school because she scored quite high on the entrance exams.

She gave up drugs in law school because she realized that she couldn't possibly pass her courses unless she did. However, she was still anxious about passing her courses and about her ability to handle the work. During the summer between her first and second years at law school, she became depressed again and was hospitalized because of suicidal thoughts. She was prescribed Zoloft in the hospital, and when she left she continued taking it under the auspices of the student health center. But she didn't pursue any psychotherapy. The Zoloft significantly diminished her sexual desire, which she actually thought was a good side effect, since it helped keep her mind on her schoolwork. She said that during law school she was a "workaholic" and did not develop any friendships or do anything except focus on her work.

Heather joined a law firm after graduating. She was very nervous about starting the job. Although she stayed on the Zoloft, she no longer felt that was sufficient for her. She was prescribed Xanax. She started taking it primarily in the morning to help calm herself before she could go to work. However, there were days when she didn't use it. She enjoyed the work at the law firm and developed an interest in personal injury law. As she was assigned cases of increasing complexity, however, she became more anxious. She started taking Xanax every day, and when she went to court she took an "extra dose" to be able to function with a veneer of calm in front of the judge and her client. Inside she was scared to death that she would forget something, that she would make a fool of herself, or that people would see that she was a fraud. At times she felt depressed and had thoughts of suicide, but these times were brief and only occurred two or three times a year. Although she enjoyed personal injury law, she began to focus on writing wills and handling estates because they involved less court work.

When one of Heather's associates saw that she was taking Xanax in the morning, he questioned her about her use. She lied and told him that she rarely took it. She did try to cut back after that but found that she was unable to because the anxiety would return so intensely. She began to have a couple of glasses of wine at night, now that she no longer had to study. Although she dated occasionally, she was terrified of getting close to anyone.

The treatment required for people with ADNOS obviously varies greatly from person to person. The severity of the anxiety, the length of time it is experienced, and the surrounding circumstances in a person's life all need to be taken into account in the treatment.

THE BENZO BLUES: THE SECONDARY FEATURES

The people I've described in this chapter and millions of others like them became mired in the Benzo Blues after they began to experience anxiety that overwhelmed them. Although the specific anxiety disorder and the individual circumstances vary so much that each person appears to be struggling with a different problem, all are physically or psychologically dependent on benzodiazepines, all are chronically anxious, and all have impaired functioning. In addition to the three main features of the Benzo Blues, they also experience other thoughts, feelings, and behaviors that are characteristic of people who become dependent on this class of drugs. Each of these secondary features occurs in many but not all people with the Benzo Blues. Let's look at these in more detail.

Benzos Provide Relief

When people who develop the Benzo Blues take their first pill, they invariably feel a sense of enormous relief. Overwhelmed by anxiety and lacking the internal resources to withstand its unpleasant sensations, they look for some external support. Each time they take a pill they continue to experience that relief. The intensity of the relief is dependent upon the severity of the anxiety, the length of time that the person has endured it, and whether or not the person has used other methods to help ameliorate it.

Most people, however, do not experience such profound relief from taking benzodiazepines. They may find the drugs helpful for a few days or so to help them get through a traumatic event such as a death in the family, but their experiences in life give them the confidence to know they can overcome adversity, and they don't continue to take medication. They are aware that these drugs are habit-forming and do not want to become dependent on them. Even though the drugs may help the symptoms of their anxiety, most people for whom they are prescribed don't take them for more than one or two weeks.

Only *Benzos Provide Relief*

Many people are able to tolerate even intense anxiety by coping in a variety of ways. They may meditate, exercise, listen to soothing music, take long walks, or engage in activities like going to the movies or reading to keep their minds occupied. They may practice relaxation techniques such as deep breathing or progressive muscular relaxation. They may use other people as supports to help them to tolerate the anxiety. They may strategize or rehearse with friends or families ways of enhancing their chances of performing well for an upcoming event. They may talk over their worries with others and take comfort from the fact that other people have successfully resolved a similar problem.

People who use benzodiazepines chronically, however, generally don't know any other effective ways of managing anxiety. They may have been able to get through other difficult situations in their lives without having been aware of their anxiety, and thus the experience of anxiety may feel quite new to them. When they first experience symptoms of anxiety, therefore, they may have had no practice with ways of coping like relaxation techniques, engaging in physical activity, sharing their feelings with friends, or even consulting a therapist. This lack of useful alternatives can lead them to seek out medication.

Daily Use

At some point the vast majority of people who use benzodiazepines regularly begin taking them daily. This may occur from the first day if that is how the drug is prescribed. But sometimes when the initial prescription is to take it "as needed," a person can gradually drift into daily use over a matter of weeks or months.

Sometimes even people who do not use benzodiazepines every day become psychologically dependent on them. These people feel that they can manage anxiety-provoking situations—as long as they know they can take a pill when they want. Such people commonly carry one or two around with them as a way of making sure that they have something that can help them if their anxiety does become overwhelming.

Most people who use benzodiazepines regularly do not escalate their dose, as can be seen with users of alcohol or narcotics. In part, this is because, unlike alcohol and narcotics, these drugs do not appear to speed up their own metabolic breakdown when they are taken regularly, therefore, a person does not need higher and higher amounts to compensate for the faster breakdown. Another important factor is that most regular users restrict their activity in order to minimize the intensity of the anxiety. Since these people limit the stress on themselves, they do not need an increased dosage.

Unsuccessful Tapering

Generally, when someone has been using a benzodiazepine regularly for some months, he or she tries to get off it. They may feel guilty about depending on a drug that they know is habit-forming, or they may want to put all their problems behind them and see the drug as a visible reminder that they haven't. Or their doctor may suggest it, knowing that the drugs are habit-forming and feeling uncomfortable about helping a patient maintain a physical dependency. These attempts are generally unsuccessful, however, due to physical dependence, psychological dependence, and the fact that the original cause of anxiety remains unresolved.

Plateau

People experience a "plateau" when they have been using benzodiazepines for many months. During this period of time the anxiety continues, although the severity may wax or wane, but the drug use continues as well. The person continues to feel anxiety, but the medication provides temporary relief. Day to day, she continues to be preoccupied with anxiety and uses any way possible to minimize it. This is a time when most people say that the medication continues to help them and they absolutely need it. They stay on the same dose during this time.

This plateau may go on for months or even years. Several unsuccessful attempts to taper the medication may take place during this time. Sometimes a physician will refuse to prescribe the drug indefinitely, but the patient then goes to a different physician to continue the prescription.

During this period of time, people often experience what Barbara Gordon, in her famous book, *I'm Dancing As Fast As I Can* called the "Scarlett O'Hara Syndrome," after that heroine's propensity to put off problems until another day. Gordon felt that when she was taking Valium, she was saying to herself, "I can't think about that now, I'll have to deal with it tomorrow."[8] The problem for Scarlett O'Hara, and for other people who take these drugs chronically, is that tomorrow doesn't come because each new day becomes another day to take the pills.

Use of Other Drugs

People afflicted by the Benzo Blues frequently use other drugs like caffeine, tobacco, and alcohol. One reason that they may need coffee to wake up is because they are somewhat oversedated from the benzodiazepine, although it is hard for them to see that connection. After a couple of cups of coffee they feel awake, but for the rest of the day they are somewhat anxious because the coffee has made them jittery. This also happens with tobacco use. The simultaneous use of alcohol and benzodiazepines is complex and is addressed in chapter 12.

People who abuse a variety of drugs such as cocaine, amphetamines, opiates, and others certainly can abuse these drugs as well. For these people, benzodiazepine use is part of a much larger problem in which they use many different substances for kicks, thrills, and as tools to alter any unpleasant feeling.

Avoiding New Activities

Because people with the Benzo Blues restrict their activities and avoid situations in which they may become anxious, they do not pursue opportunities that would allow them to develop meaningful and satisfying lives. Chief among the missed benefits is the development of new relationships, which leaves anxiety sufferers lonely and depressed. The lack of involvement with people and activities leads to other habits that may not be particularly satisfying and constructive. For example, people may stay home a lot and watch excessive amounts of television, leading to further isolation and loss of opportunities.

In short, the original problem of restricting activities because of anxiety grows into a restrictive, almost suffocating lifestyle in which there are no new opportunities. As a person's life becomes increasingly unsatisfying, he has even less motivation to pursue tasks that, although difficult, might bring more satisfaction. The motivation to taper the benzodiazepines and tolerate anxiety decreases even further.

Withdrawing from Life

Many people who suffer from anxiety or panic attacks begin to structure their lives to minimize the intensity and frequency of the symptoms of anxiety. For people with panic attacks, this may happen very early on as they attempt to minimize the likelihood of experiencing a panic attack. People with agoraphobia experience withdrawal from ongoing outside activities as perhaps the most prominent outcome of their anxiety. In people with other forms of anxiety, however, this withdrawal doesn't happen immediately and can be more subtle. As they stay on benzodiazepines over an extended period and feel increasingly unable to cope with the stresses that life presents them, their circle of contacts and experiences gradually becomes smaller and more restricted.

Troubled Relationships with Others

For people with the Benzo Blues, relationships with others are often profoundly altered. Many people who regularly use benzodiazepines tend to isolate themselves. Because these people often are able to provide little response or reciprocity their casual friendships with acquaintances tend to drop off. However, the sufferers are often quite involved with one or two people—they often experience themselves as being dependent on these friends or family members to help them manage the stresses in their life.

Increased Visits to Physician

Regular users have numerous physical complaints and more health problems,[9] which lead them to visit physicians more frequently than the average person. Sometimes the complaints can appear to be genuine physical problems. For example, with the improvements in technology and the availability of cardiac catheterization, it is apparent that many people with chest pain have normal hearts and are instead suffering from anxiety. The diagnosis of noncardiac chest pain has recently been added to the medical lexicon to describe people whose chest pain is due to anxiety. Sometimes people complain of feelings of "dizziness," "light-headedness," "stiffness," and other vague complaints that have no medical origin.

There are many reasons why people who take benzodiazepines may make more visits to their physicians. People with chronic anxiety may experience a worsening of their physical health. Also, people commonly seek prescriptions to lessen their anxiety at the same time that they address other medical problems. Some people with the Benzo Blues are unaware of what is making them anxious. Many have not developed the insight to know what they are feeling and the vocabulary to describe it. Since it is often difficult for them to articulate what exactly is distressing them psychologically, they may find it easier to seek help from a doctor by presenting a physical problem. Many users go to physicians before they will see mental health providers for help in alleviating their distress because they are reluctant to face the issues that are leading them to feel anxious.

It is important to note that some patients who stop their benzodiazepines make many fewer visits for medical services.[10]

Depression

Some people who take benzodiazepines warrant a diagnosis of clinical depression. This refers to a cluster of feelings of despair, hopelessness, tearfulness, lack of energy, and an inability to experience pleasure, and may include physical symptoms of insomnia, decreased appetite and weight loss, and even thoughts of suicide.

Sometimes the depression starts even before a person ever takes their first benzodiazepine, and the symptoms of anxiety are actually part of a depressive episode that has not been properly diagnosed. Other people gradually become depressed while they take their drugs. There is no definitive medical understanding why this happens. Do benzodiazepines cause depression as a direct effect on the brain in a manner similar to alcohol? Or is the depression more the result of life's problems gradually getting a person down?

My own belief is that these drugs cause depression for both reasons. They definitely impair a person's ability to manage life effectively, and this can certainly contribute to depression. The drugs contribute to depression as a direct effect as well. First, they diminish the intensity of feelings in everyone who takes them, and this state is also a common symptom of depression. Second, the vast majority of regular users lack a certain joie de vivre, which is also a symptom of a low-level chronic depression. Third, most people notice an increased intensity of many of their feelings, not just anxiety, as they start to taper their drug usage.

No matter what anxiety disorder a person starts with, the ongoing use of benzodiazepines gradually shapes their life in the downward spiral of the three main features of the Benzo Blues and some or all of the secondary symptoms. This spiral can start insidiously because the effect of the first dose can provide such relief that a person keeps looking for that same relief. The longer that people stay on these drugs, however, the more they begin to experience their life as a never-ending cycle of anxiety and relief. They stop taking charge of their lives and let the avoidance of anxiety be the compass that guides them. Shaping their life to maximize relief and minimize anxiety, they stay on their pills and narrow their lives. They avoid old problems and new opportunities and retreat into a superficial engagement with life.

Which features you experience depends to a great extent on the details of your makeup and personality, how long you have used the medication, and other treatment methods you may be using. Most people who are given benzodiazepines, however, do not become dependent on them. What is different about them and their experience of anxiety that leads to dependency? To answer this question, it is necessary to understand both normal and pathological anxiety, the focus of the next chapter.

· 3 ·

UNDERSTANDING NORMAL AND PATHOLOGICAL ANXIETY

Anxiety is something we all feel at different times in our lives when we experience some stress. We may experience anxiety when we worry about making a good impression on someone whom we are about to meet, when we wonder if we will beat the traffic on the way home from work, when we are concerned about whether our children will finish their homework, and during a hundred other daily events. Larger issues, such as whether we will be able to maintain or improve our financial situation, whether we will keep our jobs, or whether our relationships are satisfying obviously stress us more. We may become anxious when events occur unexpectedly and we are unsure what will happen. A death in the immediate family, development of serious physical illness, a car accident, being fired, or learning that your partner has decided to leave you can cause intense anxiety.

NORMAL ANXIETY

There are four separate parts to the experience of anxiety: thoughts, emotions, physical sensations, and behavior.

Anxious *thoughts* can range from realistic concern over day-to-day details to inappropriate preoccupation with unrealistic possibilities. Normal anxious thoughts are usually confined to the issue that is the source of the person's concern, such as getting to an appointment on time, keeping a job, getting married, or maintaining health. Anxious thoughts can be normal or pathological, de-

71

pending on the intensity and frequency with which they occur. For example, some people are sticklers for details and feel some anxiety unless everything in their home is arranged properly or all their work is done before they go to bed. For some this just means they like a neat home; for others it may mean a slavish preoccupation with cleanliness that rules their life. Anxious thoughts that are clearly pathological include concerns about things that are highly unlikely, such as Susan's worry that she might be having a heart attack, or totally unrealistic, such as Peter's obsession that he would contract AIDS from casual contact. People think the world may end or they may die or they may think that something terrible is going to happen but have no specific worry, just impending thoughts of doom.

The primary *emotion* that is present in anxiety is clearly fear, but the two are not identical. One difference is that anxiety involves a thought process that is not activated in true fear. Anxiety also contains other emotions that are absent in pure fear. For example, though anxiety itself is generally experienced as an unpleasant and negative emotion, interest and excitement can also be present when anxiety is experienced in relation to something that may turn out positively. Similarly, discouragement and depression are components of anxiety when the outcome appears negative. Finally, anxiety sometimes occurs when the threat is to a person's psychological rather than physical well-being and there is no actual danger present. For example, people can be anxious that others might not like their appearance or that their lover will leave them, though neither of these anxieties implies a bodily threat.

When mild, the *physical* sensation of anxiety is an inner feeling of uneasiness. When more severe, this sensation may be quite intense. Other physical sensations may include shortness of breath, dizziness or feelings of unsteadiness, palpitations, sweating, choking, an uncomfortable sensation in the stomach that may include nausea and even vomiting, numbness or tingling sensations, flushing or hot flashes, and chest pain.

Motor *behavior* is generally racheted up when people are anxious. Though this increase can be limited to an increased rate of breathing, a tremor, or mild restlessness, sometimes people also bite their nails, twirl their hair, wring their hands, or even pace the floor when anxious. Insomnia is not uncommon.

Is it normal to be anxious at times? What is the role of anxiety in a person's life? Does it have any useful purpose? To answer these questions fully, it would be necessary to know how the body produces the constellation of thoughts, emotions, sensations, and behaviors that constitute the experience of anxiety. Unfortunately, we know next to nothing about how the body produces thoughts and emotions. And although we understand very well how we make our muscles move, this knowledge provides little useful information about anxiety. The examination of how our body produces the physical sensations of anxiety is all that remains. Thankfully, our knowledge of these physical processes provides a clue.

The bewildering array of sensations that occurs during the experience of anxiety may seem totally unrelated. In order to explain how and why a person would feel so many physical sensations at the same time it is necessary to understand how the body, male or female, organizes all its systems.

The brain exerts control through a complex network of nerves that connect the brain to all the rest of the body. The entire apparatus is called the nervous system. The individual cells of the brain, called neurons, communicate with one another in order to insure that the body is controlled in an orderly fashion. This occurs as follows: One nerve cell "fires" and releases its chemical messenger, called a neurotransmitter, from its axon, or tail. Some chemicals that have been identified as neurotransmitters include norepinephrine, serotonin, and dopamine. The neurotransmitter traverses the space, or synapse, to the main body of an adjacent, postsynaptic neuron. The neurotransmitter makes the postsynaptic neuron either more or less likely to fire its own neurotransmitter. The anatomical organization of the brain is incredibly complex, and a single neuron receives messages from many other neurons. Depending on the sum of all the messages received, the postsynaptic neuron either fires and releases its neurotransmitter or remains quiescent. The entire brain is a series of interconnected loops of cells that affect one another; there is no "master" cell.

The brain communicates with the rest of the body through connections to the spinal cord and peripheral nerves. The portion of the nervous system called the *autonomic nervous system* is the most important in understanding the physical symptoms of anxiety. This system connects the internal organs, such as the eyes, heart, lungs, intestines, genitals, and even blood vessels, with nerves that are connected to and receive their "orders" from nerve cells in the brain and spinal cord, and regulates, among other processes, the heart rate, blood pressure, speed of digestion, and dilation of the pupils.

The autonomic system contains two separate groups of nerve cells called the *sympathetic division* and the *parasympathetic division*. The workings of these two systems together allow the body to respond to changing conditions. This is possible because the sympathetic and parasympathetic systems tend to have opposing effects. For example, the sympathetic division speeds up the heart rate, while the parasympathetic portion tends to slow it down. Each organ is able to adapt to changing circumstances in the environment by maintaining a balance of these two opposing forces.

All parts of the body make a coordinated response to the environment because the sympathetic and parasympathetic systems influence all of the body's functions. For example, when a person is exercising, the hormone adrenaline, released by the adrenal glands, will cause the sympathetic system to dominate. When this happens, we see an increase in the heart rate and more blood pumped to the muscles, faster breathing and an expansion of the lungs so that more oxygen gets in, a halting of the contractions in the bowel that aid in digestion in order to conserve energy for exercise, a narrowing of the blood vessels that go to the skin in order to conserve oxygen for the muscles, piloerection (goose bumps), and countless other processes so that the person has an integrated response appropriate to the activity and the environment. During eating, on the other hand, the parasympathetic nervous system dominates and the physical responses are very different: The mouth produces excess salivation in anticipation of food, bowel movements increase to help digest the food, the heart rate slows down, the skin relaxes so that there are no goose bumps, blood flow to the muscles decreases, and so on.

The relative dominance of either system is determined by neurons in the central nervous system. The neurotransmitter changes the balance of the sympathetic and parasympathetic divisions, altering the body's functions. Thus the physical consequence of a certain action or experience is a coordinated response of all the organ systems, allowing the body as a whole to provide the best response.

What is the characteristic response of the body during anxiety?

There is a decreased blood flow to the skin, so that the skin turns cold and clammy. Hair stands on end and goose bumps occur. Increased sweating maintains normal temperature. Dilation of the pupils enhances vision of distant objects. Decreased saliva production in the mouth preserves fluid and avoids energy waste on digestion. Movements of the upper digestive tract that usually push food through during digestion are decreased, leading to nausea and sometimes vomiting. Increased movements of the lower digestive tract lead to an increased urge to defecate. Airways in the lungs are expanded and the rate of breathing increases so that more oxygen is inhaled. An increased heart rate leads to more oxygen being pumped to the muscles. A decreased blood flow to the genitals preserves the blood supply's oxygen for other organs.

This constellation of sensations and physical changes is remarkably similar to the fight-flight response instinctive to many mammals. The response is the term given to the physiological response of animals who are under attack and must do one of two things to survive—fight or flee. Their bodies gear up to respond to the attack by focusing all their energy and systems on defending themselves.

In sum, *anxiety is a coordinated group of thoughts, emotions, sensations, and behaviors that prepare a person to respond to a perceived threat.* It is a *normal and useful response* that we all need in order to function.

PATHOLOGICAL ANXIETY

The sensations of anxiety are usually mild and limited in duration, although most of us have had a few experiences in our lives that caused intense anxiety. Some people, however, experience "pathological" anxiety—i.e., an anxiety disorder, which occurs when the sensations of anxiety are excessively intense, last longer than the situation warrants, or cause significant impairment in functioning. Although normal anxiety can be unpleasant, pathological anxiety is extremely distressing.

Anxiety disorders cause varying symptoms. Some people are plagued more by thoughts, others by physical sensations. Some people experience anxiety continuously, others for only brief periods. Some people experience anxiety as a sudden attack, while for others it builds gradually. Some people know what makes them anxious; others feel that their anxiety has no cause. Anxiety causes some people limitations in many areas of their life, but others are limited in only one or two areas.

Although "normal" anxiety is an appropriate response to a stressful situation, the meaning and cause of pathological anxiety are not quite so clear. Is it an abnormal condition that is qualitatively different from normal anxiety, or are the two somehow related? Is there any purpose to pathological anxiety? An enormous body of work addresses this question. Most researchers have confined themselves to one of three areas—the biological, psychological, and social theories of anxiety disorders.

Biological Theory

Many investigators have proposed theories that emphasize the biological makeup of pathological anxiety. Chief among these is David Sheehan, a psychiatrist who wrote *The Anxiety Disease*, a book that explores the understanding and treatment of panic disorder, who stated: "the central problem here [anxiety] springs from some source inside the individual's body, rather than a response to a situation outside the person. . . . In this anxiety disease, as in all diseases, nature has malfunctioned in some way."[1]

Theorists who favor the biological explanation use several lines of evidence to bolster their case. First, many believe that there is a genetic component to a person's experience of anxiety, that some people are constitutionally more anxious than others. They base this belief on observations that even young babies exhibit differences in temperament, shyness, and the amount of fear they show in response to new situations,[2] on the research demonstrating that anxiety disorders appear to run in families,[3] and on the higher frequency of the heart condition known as mitral valve prolapse in people who have panic attacks. Second, administration of certain chemicals induces panic attacks in people who have experienced panic attacks in the past. This suggests that there is something "different" about people who get panic attacks. Finally, a variety of drugs appear to ameliorate the symptoms of anxiety substantially, which implies that a physical process has somehow gone wrong and can be corrected. People sometimes point to the drugs' effects on the "benzodiazepine" receptor as proof that they are improving a biological disorder.

Critics of the biological theorists disagree on all three points. Although there is no question that some people are more shy, inhibited, and fearful than others, perhaps even from birth, even genetic researchers acknowledge that there is no direct genetic evidence of genes that lead a person to be more susceptible to anxiety disorders as they age. In fact, one anxiety disorder of childhood, school phobia, has been renamed separation anxiety disorder because the problem isn't a child's innate fearfulness about school. Rather, the child and one or both of the parents are uncomfortable with the growing independence of the child.

Genetic studies on identical and fraternal twins in which one twin experienced panic attacks have yielded some tantalizing findings. Identical twins are genetically identical, while fraternal twins share only fifty percent of identical genes, the same amount of genetic material as any sister and brother. The likelihood that the second twin also experienced panic attacks was thirty-one percent if the twins were identical but zero percent if the twins were fraternal.[4] Although this finding suggests a genetic component, it also demonstrates that there must be other influences besides genetics that cause panic disorder. In sixty-nine percent of the cases, one twin experienced panic attacks and the other remained panic free even though their genes were identical.

Relatives of people with anxiety disorders have a much higher risk of anxiety disorders.[5] Although geneticists have worked out numerous modes of transmission for many physical traits and diseases, no model explains the pattern of transmission in families. Just because some families may contain more people with anxiety disorders than others doesn't prove that the disorders are genetically passed down. After all, Republicanism runs in families, too, but that doesn't mean it's genetic. Since documentation for a genetic component does exist for a variety of other disorders, such as Huntington's disease or cystic fibrosis, it is reasonable to remain skeptical of the genetic component of the biological hypothesis until definitive proof emerges.

During the late seventies and early eighties, interest was stirred by findings that many patients with panic attacks also had mitral valve prolapse. The mitral valve is one of four valves in the heart that maintain the proper flow of blood through the heart and lungs. Mitral valve prolapse (MVP) is a condition in which one of the parts of the mitral valve is "floppy," allowing blood to flow in the wrong direction. Some people with MVP experience chest pain, palpitations, and light-headedness. Later researchers, however, using more reliable diagnostic equipment such as echocardiograms, demonstrated that there was not an increased frequency of MVP in people with panic disorders.[6] It has also been demonstrated that there is no increase in anxiety disorders in people with MVP.[7]

Much research has investigated the response of panic following the administration of intravenous caffeine or lactate or inhalation of carbon dioxide only in those people who have a panic disorder. This research is often cited as "proving" that those with panic disorder have some form of constitutional difference. David Clark, a psychiatrist in England, however, found that the responses of the subjects were significantly influenced by their expectations and recall of previous experiences with induced sensations.[8] Clark states that these agents may produce panic only if the bodily sensations are interpreted in a negative way. This is likely if the subject being examined has had panic attacks in the past and associates the sensations evoked by these chemicals with the sensations that occur during a panic attack. Such a person would feel that a panic attack was on its way, become more anxious, and then have a panic attack. On the other hand, people who do not have panic disorder would not associate these sensations with panic and would not become anxious or have a panic attack. Clark suggests that it is not the agents themselves causing the panic attack but rather the person's cognitive beliefs about their internal stimuli. He demonstrated the possible validity of this hypothesis by reducing the frequency of panic attacks in people with panic disorder by explaining to the patients that hyperventilation caused panic attacks and providing training in a respiratory control technique.[9]

Intravenous administration of lactate or yohimbine in people with PTSD results in panic attacks and an intensification of other symptoms of PTSD.[10] These findings are evidence for some sort of biological abnormality in people with PTSD but demonstrates that *trauma* starts the process, not some genetic or "constitutional" difference.

Finally, the notion that successful drug therapy implies a genetic/biological abnormality is just plain poor reasoning. Although the response of the body to medication can illuminate some of the physical processes *involved* in the production of an anxiety disorder, one cannot determine the cause of a disorder by any treatment, no matter how successful. The fact that one can fix a broken leg with a cast doesn't mean that the person in question has a cast deficiency or even a bone disorder; more likely they ran into a tree while skiing. A deficiency of insulin produces the manifestations of diabetes, but that knowledge doesn't explain the cause of the insulin deficiency. So just because benzodiazepines have helped many people get a good night's sleep when they were under stress doesn't mean that they have a genetic/biological abnormality that causes a sleep disorder. The existence of the "benzodiazepine" receptor only clarifies where the drugs work in the brain, not the nature of the abnormality in anxiety disorders.

The infant observations and genetic studies remain the strongest arguments to date that there may be some genetic/biological component in some patients with an anxiety disorder. No one knows what it is yet, but that doesn't mean it doesn't exist. Even if the biological component can't yet be defined, however, there is no question that the biological treatments for anxiety—medications—have provided enormous relief to millions of people.

Psychological Theory

Researchers and clinicians working from a psychological perspective seek to understand people's feelings and behavior in terms of different mental structures of the mind. Although a good number of psychological models of anxiety have been developed, many practicing therapists who see people with anxiety disorders use Freud's concepts of the way the mind is organized. Freud was among the first to identify some of the different mental structures and postulate how they interact with one another. Generations of therapists have modified and extended his theories, but much of what Freud wrote nearly a century ago retains its explanatory power.

Freud postulated three parts to the mind: the id, the superego, and the ego. The id contains two basic drives—sexuality and aggression—that Freud felt all people possess. The superego is the part of the mind that places restraints on a person's behavior. It develops, with age, from the restrictions that are placed on a child because of the dangers of certain situations. The superego allows the person (and society) to function without being overwhelmed by the free expression of the id. The ego is the rational part of the mind that moderates between the opposing forces of the id and the superego.

Freud felt that anxiety is the body's signal that these forces are in some form of conflict. He believed that conflict between the id's wishes and the superego's prohibitions leads to anxiety. For example, a person experiencing sexual interest in another person (a wish from the id) would simultaneously experience prohibitions (from the superego) that would cause her to remember all the reasons why she shouldn't have sex. The person would experience some degree of anxiety until the rational part of the mind (the ego) had resolved the situation by deciding on a course of action (i.e., to approach or back off).

Another of Freud's contributions that continues to have some value in understanding anxiety is his theory of the unconscious— that people can think about, feel, and do things for reasons that they are not necessarily aware of. The most commonly known aspect of the unconscious is the "Freudian slip," which refers to someone saying something that he did not consciously mean to say but which reflects his actual feelings.

Many psychoanalysts feel that Freud's theories are too narrow, and that a wider variety of internal conflicts cause anxiety. Although psychoanalysts may hold different views on the exact cause of anxiety, however, most would agree with Kaplan and Sadock that anxiety is "an indication that something is disturbing the internal psychological equilibrium."[11]

The evidence that anxiety can be caused by psychological abnormalities rests on two separate bodies of evidence. First, numerous studies evaluating different forms of therapy for anxiety and other psychiatric problems have demonstrated clear and long-lasting benefits from psychotherapy to people with anxiety disorders—without making any change in their biological makeup or their life circumstances. Therapists from the time of Freud have helped millions of people with anxiety improve their functioning. Although therapists hold widely divergent beliefs about the nature of the psychological problems that cause anxiety and how psychotherapy helps, too many people have gotten better from psychotherapy alone to dismiss the psychological explanation.

Second, although therapists base their interventions on different theoretical models, there must at least be some partial truth to those models in order for therapists consistently to help people successfully. For example, the proponents of cognitive therapy believe that people who experience panic attacks tend to interpret outside events and internal sensations in the most negative way possible. They call this "catastrophizing." They point to the large number of people who go to an emergency room with palpitations and shortness of breath convinced that they are having a heart attack when in fact they are experiencing a panic attack. The aim of cognitive psychotherapy is to help the patient learn to reinterpret their inner sensations and external events more realistically. Numerous studies have documented the benefits of cognitive therapy for people with panic attacks.[12]

Some critics dismiss the psychological model out of hand. They tend to be uninformed about the documentation demonstrating the partial validity of different models of anxiety and that different forms of psychotherapy are effective. More informed critics focus on the gaps and contradictions that exist in and between different psychological models. They point to irreconcilable differences between alternative models as evidence that both models must be wrong. They also point out that psychotherapy is often ineffective. These criticisms are valid to a point—the purely psychological model is clearly insufficient to explain the intensity and severity of anxiety disorders and other forms of psychiatric distress. Nevertheless, the psychological model has been far too helpful to dismiss entirely.

Social Theory

In contrast to the psychological view that anxiety is the result of internal conflicts and the biological view that anxiety results from a "disease," social theory focuses on how symptoms of anxiety develop from experiences in the environment. There is a wide and compelling body of evidence demonstrating that experiences in life can lead to anxiety in the future.[13] Central to the social or environmental theory of anxiety is the belief that stressful experiences shape people's coping styles of managing their lives. The form, intensity, and duration of the stress, and the degree of success with which the individual copes with the stress, contribute to how the person will cope with future stressful experiences.

Consider a man who goes swimming at a beach despite the display of a red flag cautioning against strong currents. Suppose he has difficulty with the current and has to receive assistance to return to shore. It is likely that this experience will remain in his mind for years, a reminder of his anxiety about drowning. Whenever that man sees a red flag, he may feel the symptoms of anxiety even though he is not in any objective danger.

A more complex reaction evolves when the stress is not a single event but is repeated many times and evokes many feelings besides anxiety. For example, many women who were sexually abused by their fathers as children associate all men and any sexual activity with their experience of abuse. Since it's very difficult to avoid running into men and it's virtually impossible to avoid sex with them if you want to have children (notwithstanding the aids to conception devised through modern technology), many women who were the victims of sexual abuse are constantly being reminded of the abuse and constantly anxious as a result.

Learning theorists feel that the most constructive treatments help a person tolerate and overcome the anxiety by exposure to the feared situation in ways that help a person learn to tolerate it without significant anxiety. This may take the form of behavioral treatments such as biofeedback or systematic desensitization if the anxiety is due to a relatively circumscribed problem. Anxiety with a more complex etiology, such as that caused by sexual abuse, may require individual psychotherapy and medication as well.

Biopsychosocial Theory

All three approaches have produced evidence demonstrating that each contributes to the production of anxiety. Much of this literature has been comprehensively reviewed by Taylor and Arnow (1988) in *The Nature and Treatment of Anxiety Disorders*. They state that "past experience, genetic endowment, and development all influence the onset, maintenance, and exacerbation of anxiety disorders." They feel that "Anxiety is best viewed from the *biopsychosocial* [emphasis added] perspective, which posits that various systems interact in complicated ways to determine the final presentation of anxiety for a particular individual."[14]

My own view of the etiology of anxiety is derived from my training and my experience as a practicing physician. Throughout my time in medical school and my postgraduate training in psychiatry, I learned to value most those teachers who were willing to embrace the complexity inherent in attempting to understand and help people with psychiatric disorders. These were teachers who generally had their own views about people but fully acknowledged new ideas that called their beliefs into question. I was fortunate to be trained in an environment in which several different theories of personality, anxiety, and treatment were valued and taught. My fellow trainees and I commonly discussed a patient's problems in a conference with several psychopharmacologists (specialists in the use of psychiatric medication) to determine what the best medicine might be for them. We then discussed the same case with psychoanalysts, who taught us what was going on inside the person's mind; behavioral psychiatrists, who taught us some practical and enormously useful psychotherapeutic techniques; and family therapists, who helped us to understand why a certain problem was occurring in a person's life at any given time. This was uncomfortable at times because of our uncertainty about how to effectively integrate such different approaches, but it helped us to avoid the trap of believing that anyone possessed a single unifying theory that could explain and treat every problem.

Like Taylor and Arnow, I feel that the biological, psychological, and social perspectives each offer compelling evidence that demonstrates some role in the production of anxiety and anxiety disorders. I differ from their interpretation, however, because I don't believe that there can be a satisfactory unifying synthesis of the evidence at this time. We are just beginning to understand how these systems actually relate to each other. Bessel van der Kolk, a psychiatrist at Harvard Medical School, has written a series of articles exploring the biological mechanisms that underlie PTSD in veterans who have experienced wartime trauma. He has convincingly demonstrated that men who experience this trauma have alterations in the physiological regulation of their brain endorphins and that these alterations produce some of the clinical manifestations of PTSD.[15] J. D. Bremner, a psychiatrist at the West Haven, Connecticut, Veterans Hospital, has hypothesized that stress impairs short-term memory by damaging the hippocampus, an area of the brain involved in memory, by showing that veterans with PTSD had a smaller hippocampus.[16] Other theorists are working on the connections between stress, the hormone cortisol, the immune system, and physical illness but have not yet made specific connections between them. Our knowledge of the linkage between the three areas still has too many gaps that are filled with hope and theory, not fact. Even the most complete and elegant theory cannot account for the subtle differences in a person's physiology or psychology that can help us to predict how he or she will react to events in life and whether any specific anxiety disorder will develop.

Nevertheless, I believe that the biopsychosocial model is the best and most useful at the present. Even though the connections between the three elements are not well understood, the view afforded by the biopsychosocial model is sufficient to clarify that pathological anxiety is not some bizarre unexplainable illness that comes out of nowhere. Rather, it is *an abnormal process that emerges from the same experiences and biological systems that generate the process of normal anxiety.*

Regardless of how pathological anxiety arises, though, it is intensely distressing to experience and leads people to look anywhere for relief. This search for relief is not the only reason that people become dependent on benzodiazepines, however. Chapter 4 examines the roles played by five major participants in the creation and maintenance of the Benzo Blues.

✦ 4 ✦

THE FORCES THAT CREATE THE BENZO BLUES

It may seem straightforward when a doctor prescribes a benzodiazepine for anxiety. The patient is anxious, the doctor wants to help, and the patient walks out of the doctor's office with a prescription. In fact, however, the acts of writing and filling that prescription are the culmination of an array of forces: the drugs themselves, the companies that make them, the doctors who prescribe them, the patients who request them, and any third-party payer such as an insurance company. As we'll see, these drugs are prescribed for many reasons that have nothing to do with anxiety and the best treatment for an individual.

BENZODIAZEPINES

Chemical Properties

The term *benzodiazepine* refers to the chemical structure that is common to all these drugs. It consists of a *benz*ene ring of six carbon atoms connected to a seven-membered *diazepine* ring. Most benzodiazepines have an additional ring as well. Different benzodiazepines have different elements attached to the rings. These differences affect the drugs' solubility in the blood, brain, and fat tissue, and account for the different rates of absorption, metabolism, and excretion.

Benzodiazepines are sometimes referred to as sedatives or hypnotics. A sedative agent "allays excitement"—produces a calming effect—while a hypnotic agent induces sleep. Although some are

85

used primarily as sedatives and others as hypnotics, the pharmacological effects of all benzodiazepines are similar.

There is no theory that fully explains how benzodiazepines exert their complex effects on the brain. It is likely that they interact with a special protein found in some brain cells that has been termed the "benzodiazepine receptor."[1] The benzodiazepine receptor is a protein that sits in the middle of the cell membrane, or wall. Its function is to interact with neurotransmitters released from other nerve cells and other chemicals that arrive from the blood supply. Benzodiazepines interact with benzodiazepine receptors located in cells that release the neurotransmitter gamma-aminobutyric acid (GABA). GABA is found in many different areas of the brain and contributes to the brain's overall organization by inhibiting or minimizing the effects of other neurotransmitters such as norepinephrine, dopamine, and serotonin. Most evidence suggests that benzodiazepines minimize symptoms of anxiety by intensifying the effects of GABA.

Discontinuance Syndrome

If stopping use of a drug produces specific symptoms, the drug is said to produce a "discontinuance syndrome." Many drugs can produce a discontinuance syndrome, including those as commonly available as alcohol, caffeine, and tobacco. Prescription medicines that can produce this syndrome include phenobarbital and valproic acid, which are used to prevent seizures, and narcotics used for pain relief. It is now widely accepted that benzodiazepines can cause a discontinuance syndrome[2] with the usual therapeutic doses after only a few weeks of administration.[3]

A task force report of the American Psychiatric Association divides the "discontinuance syndrome" into three categories of symptoms: rebound, recurrence, and withdrawal.[4]

Rebound refers to a time-limited return of the original symptoms for which the benzo is prescribed, and in a more intense form than before treatment. For example, temazepam may help someone who has difficulty falling asleep. After it is stopped, however, there may be a few nights when the patient has even more difficulty falling asleep than before she began taking temazepam.

Recurrence, the return of symptoms, occurs when the benzos have been discontinued but the cause of the original symptoms has not been corrected. Since the symptoms of anxiety rather than its cause were treated, the symptoms return. In the example above, if the patient had insomnia because she was fired and was worried about her finances, her insomnia wouldn't improve until she either had found a new job or had otherwise come to terms with the situation. Unlike rebound symptoms, the original symptoms that recur after stopping benzos persist over time and retain their original intensity.

Rebound and recurrence symptoms can be difficult to distinguish from each other. In general, they occur together.

Withdrawal refers to the development of symptoms that a person has never experienced before. The most serious symptom that can occur when benzodiazepines are stopped is a seizure. Although seizures can occur from discontinuing a therapeutic dose of any benzodiazepine, it is more likely to occur when a high dose is abruptly discontinued. *Withdrawal seizures are a serious side effect, and no benzodiazepine should ever be stopped abruptly or without a physician's supervision.* Other symptoms of withdrawal include, but are not limited to, anxiety, insomnia, irritability, headaches, tremors, nausea, vomiting, diarrhea, mental impairment, weight loss, sweating, blurry vision, visual and auditory perceptual changes.

The severity of the symptoms varies tremendously in different individuals. Factors include the size of the daily dose, the length of time that a person has been on the drug, the speed with which the drug is metabolized in the body, and the rate at which the drug is tapered or stopped. Alcohol abusers and women tend to have more severe symptoms upon discontinuing these drugs.[5] The symptoms are generally more easily tolerated if the dosage is tapered over an extended period of time with small but steady reductions. Withdrawal symptoms generally last a matter of some weeks.

People who have been taking benzodiazepines daily for many months or years will generally experience symptoms of the discontinuance syndrome with *any* reduction in dosage size. If they try to stop taking them entirely, they will usually notice marked anxiety within a matter of twenty-four to seventy-two hours. Within several days the anxiety and the physical sensations can become overwhelming.

Most chronic users have experienced some symptoms of the discontinuance syndrome. The patient and her doctor may think that the patient is experiencing her old familiar symptoms of anxiety, unaware that some of the symptoms were due to the benzodiazepines themselves.

History

It might appear that the popularity of benzodiazepines in recent years is a new phenomenon caused by the increasing stress of the modern world. In fact, however, they have merely replaced other tranquilizers. For thousands of years, people from many different cultures have ingested substances to soothe their mental state. Myriad forms of alcohol, opiates, stimulants, and hallucinogenic drugs have been discovered, created, and used. It is not surprising, therefore, that mind-altering drugs have been widely developed as medical technology has grown in the last hundred years. From anesthetics for surgery, through opiates for the relief of pain, to hypnotics to aid in sleep, pharmaceutical creativity has known almost no bounds.

Anxiety has been a major reason for the development of mood-altering drugs. Bromide was the first agent to be introduced as a sedative back in 1853. Chloral hydrate, paraldehyde, urethane, and sulfonal were also developed in the nineteenth century for this purpose. Barbiturates, derived from barbituric acid, were introduced in the 1900s and were widely used for the first half of the century.[6] Gradually, however, problems with the use of barbiturates were recognized. Symptoms of intoxication were evident at doses that were effective for anxiety, and the drugs caused physical dependence and tolerance, a term used to describe the diminished effectiveness of a drug used regularly. Most troubling, they caused potentially lethal reactions during withdrawal or overdosage.

These difficulties led to the search for other agents by drug companies intent on expanding sales. Propanediols, which derive their name from the base chemical structure of propane, were the next group to be widely used. The most famous was Miltown which was marketed in the late fifties. Other popular agents included Quaalude, Placidyl, and Doriden. It soon became apparent, however, that these drugs shared the same undesirable effects as barbiturates.

The search for other tranquilizers continued, and in the mid-fifties Roche Laboratories developed the first benzodiazepine, chlordiazepoxide. It was almost discarded because it was initially given in excessive dosages and resulted in patients having difficulty walking and talking.[7] Eventually, however, the effective dosage range was determined, and it was marketed as Librium in 1960. Valium was released shortly thereafter and quickly became the most frequently prescribed benzodiazepine and one of the most popular drugs of all time. By 1987, Xanax had overtaken Valium.

Many people felt that drugs like Valium and Librium were addictive and more dangerous than the medical profession had acknowledged. Charlotte Muller, a professor of urban studies at the City University of New York, wrote about the excessive reliance on pills in "The Overmedicated Society: Forces in the Marketplace for Medical Care" in *Science* magazine in 1972. *The Tranquilizing of America: Pill-Popping and the American Way of Life* by Richard Hughes and Robert Brewin called attention to this same issue in 1979. In *I'm Dancing As Fast As I Can* (1979) Barbara Gordon described her addiction to Valium and the difficulties that she faced in coming off it. Congressional hearings held in 1979 documented both that doctors have a predilection for prescribing benzodiazepines and that patients experience difficulty stopping the medication. The *New York Times* quoted Senator Edward Kennedy, the chairman of the hearings, as saying, "If you require a daily dose of Valium to get you through each day, you are hooked and should seek help."[8] An article titled "Benzodiazepines: The Opium of the Masses," published in 1978 by Lader, criticized their excessive use: "It is much cheaper to tranquilize distraught housewives living in isolation in tower-blocks with nowhere for their children to play than to demolish these blocks and to rebuild on a human scale, or even to provide play-groups. The drug industry, the government, the pharmacist, the tax-payer, and the doctor all have vested interests in 'medicalizing' socially determined stress responses."[9]

The negative publicity about the side effects of sedation and physical dependence caused by benzodiazepines began to have some effect. The number of prescriptions for them gradually dropped from a high of eighty-seven million in 1973 to fifty-five million in 1981. In a study examining the effectiveness of Valium, 51 out of 119 patients who took the drug dropped out of the study because of negative publicity in the media.[10] Because both doctors and patients were realizing that benzodiazepines were more addictive than had been originally believed, it appeared that their use would continue to decrease.

The gradual disillusionment in the seventies did not spell their doom, however. Their reputation was saved as a result of two separate chains of events. The first was an unprecedented marketing campaign by Upjohn for their newest entry into the benzodiazepine market: Xanax. This campaign was unique in a number of ways and it almost singlehandedly refurbished the dwindling reputation of benzodiazepines for the treatment of anxiety. The second was a sea change in the psychiatric profession. The psychoanalysts who had been holding the upper hand for many decades in the long-running debate about the importance of intrapsychic issues in the creation of anxiety and other psychiatric disorders were gradually dethroned. Let us first look at how drug companies market their products.

THE DRUG COMPANIES

A second participant in the creation of the Benzo Blues is the pharmaceutical industry. Obviously, these companies benefit from continued prescription and administration of any medication. Some would argue that their profits depend on the development of benzodiazepines and other addictive drugs. However, drug companies benefit from the manufacture and sale of *any* drug that is popular, addictive or not. Without the financial incentive of profits, the development of many drugs that have been of considerable benefit would not have been pursued. Further, medications that were used for anxiety prior to the synthesis and distribution of benzodiazepines, such as barbiturates and propanediols like Meprobamate (Equanil, Miltown), were more addictive, more dangerous, and much less effective. But the fact remains that the pharmaceutical companies make a variety of contributions to the inappropriate use of this class of drugs.

They make the greatest profit from sales of new drugs on which they retain patents. A patent allows a drug company to be the exclusive manufacturer and seller of a new drug. Without competition in the marketplace, the company can set the price for the drug as high as it wants, thus recovering the cost of its development. But this situation prevails only while the company has the exclusive rights of the patent, currently seventeen years. Once the patent runs out, any drug company can manufacture and sell the drug. Since the new companies to enter the specific drug's market have not had to pay for its development, they can sell it at a much lower price than the original patent holder. Therefore, a company with a drug patent wants to make as much money as it can while it has exclusivity. To accomplish this, pharmaceutical companies conduct huge marketing campaigns to make the drugs for which they hold patents popular as quickly as possible. How does this work?

Pharmaceutical companies pay doctors to conduct research studies on a new drug in an effort to showcase it in the best light. If a study shows that their drug is successful, a pharmaceutical company will distribute the results of the study widely. Sometimes the company will print up the results of their study in a glossy monograph and distribute it directly to doctors at conferences or at their offices. Although the ostensible purpose is "informing" the doctor about the new drug, it's important to recognize that the drug companies present no information that is significantly negative about the drug. Nor do they disclose other studies that may demonstrate the usefulness of other medications or treatment methods for the problem.

Drug company researchers also submit their work to "independent" journals that are published by organizations such as the American Psychiatric Association. Publication in independent journals provides a veneer of "objectivity," and thus respectability, to the findings. However, there is often a subtle blurring of interests between the companies that push the drugs, the researchers who need the money to pursue their interests, and the journals that need impressive articles to enhance their reputation. When the interests of all three converge, the close relationship can dramatically slant the supposed "truth" about a drug. No journal can be entirely free of bias from the editors, researchers, and financial backers of a study, but the tremendous financial power of the drug companies buys them undue access to publicity and respectability.

Drug companies also sponsor conferences on problems that their drugs can solve. For example, a company marketing a new pain reliever may sponsor a conference on "Headaches: Their Diagnosis and Treatment." The name of the drug they are marketing is then ubiquitous—on the brochure advertising the conference, on the signs at the conference, and on the notebooks, pens, and paper that are distributed gratis. Even though many doctors are disgusted with these blatant tactics aimed at cultivating their attention and loyalty, the companies reap significant name recognition for their products. As any advertising executive from Madison Avenue knows, name recognition—whether positive or negative—increases sales.

Drug companies will pay for lunches and dinners for doctors while they are pitching their new products. I have received several offers of a hundred dollars to "participate" in teleconferences organized by drug companies, in which the only requirement is to listen on the phone to a discussion by other psychiatrists for an hour. Sales representatives continually attempt to meet with doctors in their offices in order to promote their particular drugs. In addition, pharmaceutical companies often provide free samples of their drugs to doctors in the hope that doctors will give them to patients. This gets the doctor used to prescribing the drug and patients interested in taking it. Of course, the drug is only free once; after the first time, it must be paid for.

Drug companies advertise their products in every arena possible. The *Physicians' Desk Reference (PDR)* is considered one of the major references for doctors, and is sometimes referred to as the "Bible" of drug information, but it is essentially one large advertisement. Companies buy space and give prescribing information for drugs they are promoting, but they provide no evidence in the *PDR* for their claims. Drug companies also buy advertising space in independent journals. For instance, drug companies bought more than eighty percent of the advertising space in the January 1997 issue of *The American Journal of Psychiatry,* a figure that is typical for that journal. Ads in most journals feature glossy pictures and a few brief statements trumpeting the advantages of a particular drug. In recent years, pharmaceutical companies have begun to advertise their drugs directly to the consumer in forums such as popular magazines, newspapers, and television. They know that patients will then ask their doctors about the drug regardless of whether the drug might make sense for them or not. In the advertisements any problem is reduced to a few well-chosen words, obscuring the complexity and variables inherent in almost any medical condition.

Although few doctors would prescribe anything on the basis of an advertisement, the continual bombardment of simple messages from the drug companies has the effect of shutting out other more complex and more complete messages. This has been especially true in the marketing of benzodiazepines. For example, an ad for

Restoril in the *American Journal of Psychiatry* in 1984 compares different benzodiazepines as if they were the only choice in treating insomnia and then emphasizes that the particular advantage of Restoril is its half-life. (A drug's half-life is a measure of how quickly it is metabolized by the body and gives an indication how long its effects will last.) But the ad neglects to mention that a particular patient may be using excessive caffeine, that there are other nonaddictive methods to encourage falling asleep, or that the patient could be depressed and in need of antidepressants, not just sleeping pills. Unless a doctor takes the time to question a patient closely about the issues that may contribute to the insomnia, it is only too easy to remember "Restoril, it's got the most appropriate half-life, that's what I'll prescribe." Finally, the fact that it can lead to dependency and should be used only for the short term is mentioned only in small print, on the next page.

Another way that drug companies attempt to shape doctors' thinking is to use scientific jargon and subtly distort the complexities to their advantage. For example, they often highlight the term *benzodiazepine receptor* in their ads, as if these drugs are somehow working "with" the brain, perhaps like some natural chemical. There is no evidence, however, of a "natural" benzodiazepine in the brain that normally plays this role. The advertisements thus give the false impression that these drugs were scientifically created for the express purpose of working with the body in order to minimize anxiety in the brain.

In marketing benzodiazepines, drug companies also repeatedly use the term *anxiolytic*, a combination of two words, *anxiety*, and *lysis*, which means to destroy or break up. The use of this term to describe benzodiazepines is misleading. First, it implies that anxiety is like an abscess—an uncomfortable condition that is disconnected to anything the person might be going through. It also implies that something can fix it easily. Both of these notions are false.

Marketing techniques can be so effective that doctors become convinced of the usefulness of a particular drug even when the pharmacological properties are inappropriate for the use that is pushed in the marketing. For example, Dalmane has been aggressively and successfully marketed as a sleep aid. It may give a good night's sleep for a couple of weeks, but its effects last several days. As a result, people have a significant amount in their system the next day, leading to a "hangover." Benzodiazepines with a shorter period of effectiveness are a more sensible choice.

These marketing techniques and some others were used by Upjohn in the early eighties in the most ambitious effort to date by any drug company in their effort to promote the sales of Xanax, the newest entry into the benzodiazepine market. Already approved by the FDA for general use by physicians in the treatment of anxiety, Upjohn set out to obtain FDA approval for the newly recognized panic disorder.

There were two factors that Upjohn hoped would give their latest entry an edge in the marketplace. First, Xanax (alprazolam) was marketed as one of a "new" class of benzodiazepines because of a slight modification to its chemical structure. It appeared that the new structure caused less drowsiness than other benzodiazepines, and doses high enough to stop panic attacks would not cause excessive sedation. Upjohn hoped this would increase its popularity. Second, the patent for Valium, manufactured by Roche, was due to expire in 1984. Upjohn knew that Roche would lose interest in pushing Valium after 1984 because their profits would be eaten up by companies that made a generic alternative.

Seeing a possible bonanza, Upjohn launched an unprecedented campaign to promote Xanax. They did not restrain themselves to the usual blitz of advertising, however. The company also funded one of the most ambitious studies ever undertaken on any drug, the Cross-National Collaborative Panic Study (CNCPS). The aim and scope of the CNCPS were described by Gerald Klerman, M.D., the chief investigator of CNCPS, a member of the Department of Psychiatry at Cornell University Medical School in New York and nationally known researcher and clinician, in an article that preceded the presentation of the first results of the CNCPS in the *Archives of General Psychiatry*, an official journal of the American Medical Association.[11]

He related that in the summer of 1982, Upjohn initiated a research program to evaluate the efficacy of alprazolam for panic disorder. The company then hosted a conference on anxiety in December 1982 to which they brought more than a hundred experts in the field of anxiety. Klerman reported that the decision to proceed with clinical trials of Xanax was made at this conference. The first phase of their ambitious plan compared Xanax and placebo in over five hundred patients for eight weeks at eight institutions in the United States, Canada, and Australia. Phase II took place at twelve different centers in North America, South America, and Western Europe from 1984 to 1986 and compared Xanax, placebo, and imipramine (Tofranil). The results of Phase I were reported in the May 1988 issue of the *Archives of General Psychiatry* in three separate articles. The conclusion of the first phase of the CNCPS was reported by Ballenger in the first of the three articles in the *Archives*: "Alprazolam was found to be effective and well tolerated."[12]

Many people have criticized the CNCPS, however. One major criticism was that the researchers had lost their scientific objectivity because of their close involvement with Upjohn. Although Gerald Klerman was identified only as a member of the Cornell Department of Psychiatry in his introduction to the CNCPS, contrarian psychiatrist Peter Breggin states that Klerman was, in fact, a paid consultant to Upjohn from 1982 or 1983 on.[13] His disingenuous "introduction," then, rather than being an objective review by a highly respected research clinician, is like an endorsement, similar to that of a basketball star promoting a certain brand of sneakers.

Perhaps of even greater concern is that Daniel X. Freedman, the editor in chief of the *Archives* for more than twenty years and lead author of the three-volume classic *Comprehensive Textbook of Psychiatry, also* served as a consultant to Upjohn to oversee patient safety and maintenance of the protocol. It is troubling that Freedman would place himself in a position with such an obvious conflict of interest. It strains credulity to imagine that one could get unbiased information about Xanax from a journal whose editor in chief serves as a consultant to Upjohn. Reading the study in the *Archives* is like reading studies about cigarettes and lung cancer funded by tobacco companies.

Not only the senior investigator and editor in chief at the *Archives* had ties to Upjohn, however. In their review of the marketing of Xanax, *Consumer Reports* quotes Isaac Marks, author of *Fears, Phobias, and Rituals*, as saying that "the most senior psychiatrists in the world were . . . flooded with offers of consultancies," i.e., they were paid to be part of the study.[14] Upjohn sponsored conferences on drug treatment for panic disorder and then invited its consultants to speak. Because so many clinicians were involved in the study itself, the alleged effectiveness of Xanax for panic could be communicated informally throughout the psychiatric world long before the results of the study were actually available for peer review.

Upjohn's sponsorship of the CNCPS was enormously effective. By 1987, Xanax was the most frequently prescribed benzodiazepine of all, a year before any data from the CNCPS was published. Upjohn had been able to capture the market before the data had been officially presented to the general medical community.

The exposure of Upjohn's close ties to researchers, consultants, and the editor in chief of the *Archives* as well as the flaws in the study itself (described in the appendix), came far too late to have any detrimental effect on the popularity of Xanax. It was approved by the FDA for panic disorder in 1990. The rise of the "biological" revolution in psychiatry and the marketing of Xanax by Upjohn had largely drowned out dissenting voices that opposed the long-term use of Xanax.[15] Benzodiazepines have enjoyed a poplar reputation ever since.

The only concrete action to address the overuse of benzodiazepines has been taken by the New York state legislature. It enacted a law in 1989 that required a copy of all prescriptions for benzodiazepines to be filed with the New York Department of Health. This law resulted in a thirty-to-sixty-percent reduction in the amount of benzodiazepines prescribed between 1988 and 1989 as measured by IMS America, Medicaid, and Blue Cross/Blue Shield.[16] It also resulted in a reduction in emergency admissions in New York state for overdose of the drugs from 2,637 in 1988 to 1,617 in 1989.[17]

The lack of awareness about the political and financial machinations that led to the approval of Xanax by the FDA continues to this day. One patient even told me that Xanax was necessary to fix "a benzodiazepine deficiency." Physicians have referred people to me for treatment of their anxiety after changing them from Valium to Xanax "because Xanax is the only drug that is approved by the FDA for panic disorder."

THE DOCTOR

In medical school, physicians are taught in staggering detail about the body and how it works in both sickness and health. The purpose behind medical education is simple and plain—to alleviate human suffering. The main reason that physicians prescribe benzo-diazepines, then, is the same reason that they recommend any other kind of treatment: to relieve that suffering. But when patients complain of anxiety to a physician, a number of factors may interfere with a complete evaluation and recommendations for comprehensive treatment of their pain.

THE MODEL OF ANXIETY

The major factor that influences physicians' use of these drugs is their theoretical understanding of anxiety. Sigmund Freud was one of the first physicians to construct a model of anxiety and propose a treatment derived from it. Freud believed that anxiety resulted solely from intrapsychic conflict. His innovation of "talking therapy" in the early 1900s helped many people with different forms of anxiety. His theories and methods grew in popularity among psychiatrists and spread to this country after World War II. Psychoanalysts became the most prestigious subgroup of psychiatrists because their theories of personality were all-encompassing and appeared to have enormous validity, and their treatments clearly helped many people. Psychoanalysis, with its four or five weekly sessions with the patient facing away from the analyst, proved impractical for large numbers of patients, but modifications including less frequent sessions and talking face-to-face to the therapist allowed many people to benefit. As the fifties and sixties progressed, more and more people sought help from psychotherapists.

The main problem was that psychoanalysts thought they could explain *everything* by means of examining a person's internal conflicts. Not only did they believe their theories could explain patently psychiatric problems, but they also held that such medical illnesses as asthma and ulcerative colitis were simply manifestations of intrapsychic conflict. The strength of their beliefs was such that they rarely published comparison studies with sufficient numbers of patients receiving a different treatment from psychoanalysis, such as medication.

Many psychiatrists had long thought that the psychoanalytic view was far too limited. They questioned the validity of a theory that was based on little more than anecdotal reports. The lack of solid scientific studies by analysts became increasingly unsatisfactory to the psychiatric community as a whole. In the late sixties and early seventies, increasing numbers of psychiatrists began to argue that more rigorous scientific work was needed to provide the foundation for the understanding and treatment of psychiatric disorders.

These psychiatrists succeeded in grabbing the reins of power in the psychiatric community in the late seventies. Their influence was crucial in changing the purpose, tone, and content of the publication of the third volume of the American Psychiatric Association's *Diagnostic and Statistical Manual-III*, or *DSM-III*, in 1980. Where the previous manual had been relatively loose in its definitions of different disorders and often drew upon views of intrapsychic conflict derived from psychoanalytic theory that had never been rigorously validated, *DSM-III* tried a new approach. Gone was the emphasis on intrapsychic conflict. All disorders were now rigorously defined by objective criteria that everyone could understand. Anxiety disorders were now defined as a collection of outward manifestations of specific symptoms, rather than by observation of intrapsychic conflict by trained analysts. For example, panic disorder, defined primarily on the basis of panic attacks, was no longer subsumed under the term *anxiety neurosis* but appeared as a separate anxiety disorder.

This new way of viewing anxiety led to an explosion of research that illuminated many aspects of anxiety. Now that diagnostic categories were more narrowly defined, researchers could study populations that were truly homogeneous. They would no longer study a hodgepodge of people who were diagnosed with "chronic anxiety."

This new way of viewing psychiatric disorders was used by David Sheehan, M.D., a Harvard psychiatrist, in his book *The Anxiety Disease* (1983) to explain what *DSM-III* and *DSM-IV* call panic disorder.[18] He described panic attacks as "endogenous" anxiety, meaning that the symptoms are produced within a person and are not a response to external events. He stated that the body has "malfunctioned" in a manner similar to other medical diseases. He emphasized the evidence that supported the theory that anxiety is due to biological abnormalities.

Sheehan recommended medication as the prime mode of treatment for panic attacks. He stated that many people need no other treatment, although he acknowledged that people with more severe symptoms may need behavioral therapy. He described three kinds of drugs that can provide some benefit. He quickly disparaged the first, drugs like imipramine and phenelzine that are also used as antidepressants, by stating that they are "disruptive," "unpleasant," and ineffective for the first several weeks. He then dismissed the beta-blockers such as propanolol as ineffective as well. But he advocated Xanax, describing it as less "disruptive" with fewer side effects, and mentioned drowsiness as the only one.

Sheehan described panic disorder better than anyone else had until that point. He accurately described its salient symptoms and effects over the course of a person's life, differentiated it from other illnesses, framed a believable theoretical understanding of its causes, and provided a coherent and useful treatment program to help people with the distress it causes.

Sheehan was not the only psychiatrist in the seventies and eighties to emphasize the biological underpinnings and treatment of a psychiatric disorder. New research into schizophrenia, manic-depressive disorder (now called bipolar disorder), autism, and depression documented that these disorders, too, often had some genetic basis, had characteristic physical abnormalities that could be demonstrated in the laboratory or on an X ray, and could be improved through medication. The performance of increasingly solid research appeared to be leading the field to the understanding that *all* psychiatric disorders were biologically based. This change came to be called the "biological revolution" in psychiatry.

The increasing number of people who believed in this revolution ignored Sheehan's careful effort to distinguish between when he was relaying evidence and when he was promoting a theory. His proposition that panic disorder is a "disease" became a "fact" that took on a life of its own. Physicians increasingly came to believe that panic disorder was a psychiatric problem that had no relationship to any external events. The psychoanalysts who had emphasized the careful, and slow, exploration of a patient's inner thoughts and feelings to help cure them of anxiety were left behind. In their place, physicians and patients alike sought rapid relief through drug therapy, which became the primary treatment recommended for people with anxiety.

Though incomplete, the biological model provided the intellectual foundation for physicians to choose drugs as their first option for treatment. Other factors influence physicians' reliance as well.

Time

Emergency room physicians are often the first to see someone suffering from anxiety, usually a panic attack. Their role is to provide quick relief, and they rarely have the time or the inclination to perform a full evaluation of a person's anxiety. They treat the problem with a benzodiazepine, knowing it will calm the patient down—and then move on to the next patient.

Another group of physicians that commonly sees people when they first complain of anxiety are internists, and general and family practitioners, commonly referred to as primary care providers. While it is common practice to fully investigate the sources of any physical symptoms, many primary care providers fail to adequately investigate all the sources of a patient's anxiety. The process of sorting out the sources of anxiety involves exploring a number of possibilities and areas of a person's life. This process can be quite involved and can take a significant amount of time. Partly because of financial concerns, the average primary care physician does not schedule more than fifteen or twenty minutes for a routine visit, which is not nearly enough time to perform an adequate assessment of a person's anxiety.

Lack of Training about Psychiatric Disorders

Primary care providers write most benzodiazepine prescriptions.[19] Unfortunately, most of them have not received sufficient training to perform a complete psychiatric evaluation. Their exposure to psychiatric illnesses and treatments is generally limited to several weeks of working with a few patients. They commonly prescribe this class of drugs in spite of their limited knowledge, however, because they think they are at least being somewhat helpful.[20]

Not uncommonly, benzodiazepines are prescribed for symptoms of anxiety when the patient is actually suffering from depression.[21] This unfortunate occurrence causes the patient to be exposed to the harmful effects of these drugs, and the depression remains untreated.

Anxiety As Symptom, Not Signal

Most physicians don't investigate anxiety as fully as they might because they view anxiety primarily as an unpleasant group of symptoms to be taken away as soon and as completely as possible. Many believe the common misconception that anxiety can "come out of the blue" and that a detailed evaluation is unnecessary. This is a fundamental misconception of the role that anxiety plays in a person's life. Anxiety is a sign that external events are threatening, and to cope successfully, the person needs to respond to those events. Prescribing benzodiazepines prevents that signal from being heard and interferes with the patient's responding successfully.

Lack of Familiarity with Other Treatment Methods

Some doctors prescribe benzodiazepines because they have not familiarized themselves with other methods of managing anxiety. For example, exposure therapy, in which a person confronts a feared situation, is a very effective treatment for agoraphobia.[22] Yet physicians rarely recommend it, seldom going beyond a cursory suggestion to the patient to "get out as much as you can." Similarly, short-term group therapy that focuses on relaxation techniques has been shown to be as effective for insomnia as benzodiazepines.[23] However, most primary care physicians have very little knowledge of these treatment methods.

Asking Questions Makes People More Anxious

One of the deterrents to pursuing a full investigation about the sources of a patient's anxiety is that questioning often makes him or her feel even more nervous, at least initially. Asking a lot of questions about specific problems and how they developed may make her feel even worse. The physician who glosses over the details by quickly giving a prescription makes her feel better both at the moment and then later when she takes the medication, even though the problem remains untouched.

Giving Pills Fits the Medical Model

Writing a drug prescription fits in with the general medical model, in which every problem has at least a partial physiological solution. Most physicians try to "do something" for a patient who seeks their aid. They are used to giving people medication as a way of alleviating suffering. This can be a hard reflex to break. Not prescribing medication makes many doctors feel that they haven't helped. It goes against the grain for most doctors to see that the only true solution to the symptoms of anxiety comes from within a person's own capacities, not from external aids.

If People Ask, It's Difficult to Withhold a "Helpful" Treatment

Doctors often give benzodiazepines because patients ask for them, saying they've been helpful. It doesn't take years of practice to figure out that when people complain of any symptoms of anxiety, the prescription of a benzodiazepine will bring expressions of gratitude. This is especially true for people who use the drugs regularly. Regular users will sometimes try any argument that has a chance of working in order to stay on them. Patients can become furious and even physically intimidating if they are refused. Some patients tell the doctor that they will go out and use drugs off the street or get drunk if they are not given a prescription. Some patients will even state that they feel they may kill themselves if the drugs are not prescribed. It can be hard for a physician to resist when patients are insistent, saying that "benzos are the only thing that helps"—and when patients feel so satisfied.

It is interesting to note that these are some of the same arguments that some people use in order to obtain narcotics. Most physicians are aware that the regular use of narcotics is unwise. Somehow, however, this lesson has not been applied to benzodiazepines.

Many doctors may feel uncomfortable refusing to give a person medication for anxiety if the person directly requests it. Physicians feel that they are withholding an aid that a person is reasonably seeking. They may be troubled about the general problem of dependence on benzodiazepines, but the patient in front of them is in pain *now* and needs help.

"Special Patients"

Sometimes the person requesting benzodiazepines is a patient who is important to the physician in some context other than the doctor/patient relationship. In small communities physicians know people in a variety of roles. A doctor may be treating people who are relatives of other physicians he knows and works with, who work in the hospital, with whom he has other dealings in the town or in business. This association may lead to a wish to cover up sources of anxiety in order to help the person function, rather than trying to uncover the sources of anxiety so that he can work on solving the real problem.

Whatever the reasons, the fact is that doctors may help patients stay mired in the Benzo Blues, even though their goal was only to help.

PATIENTS

Many people are susceptible to developing dependence on benzodiazepines even before they are prescribed. Some think that any intense negative emotion, such as anxiety or anger, is somehow inappropriate or that there is something wrong with them if they experience such emotions. In childhood their parents may have communicated that experiencing or expressing some strong feelings is inappropriate. For example, many parents blithely tell children not to worry about certain experiences, such as starting a new grade in school. In fact, it is natural for a child to be worried about such things, but he soon gets the message that feelings of anxiety should be ignored or denied. Such people may not understand that the emotions of anxiety, distress, sadness, and sleeplessness are normal in some situations. This can lead them to seek out medication in an effort to have their reasonable symptoms taken away.

In addition, taking drugs to improve our lives is part of the fabric of our society. Whether it's chemotherapy for cancer, antibiotics for pneumonia, ibuprofen for headaches, herbs and vitamins for "natural" ways to improve our health, or nicotine, alcohol, and marijuana for fun, we have all participated, in one fashion or another, in the pharmacological supermarket that is currently available in the modern world. Most of us know that this market contains "tranquilizers" and that these drugs are supposed to help people if they are feeling distressed. We may have heard about these drugs from television, newspapers, or family and friends. Some of us may have taken them before. Many people, therefore, go to the doctor with the expectation that he or she can and should give them a drug that will take their unpleasant symptoms away. I have been approached in one of three ways.

Demanders

Some people demand that they be given benzodiazepines for symptoms of anxiety. Generally, these patients have taken one of these drugs before, so they know that the drugs will calm them down. Demanders are generally uninterested in hearing that there is any downside to taking these drugs and focus only on the relief that is just a prescription away. These people do not want to listen to any argument or warning about the negative long-term consequences. (In fact, they may already be experiencing the Benzo Blues from their past use.) They may use a variety of arguments—of questionable validity—in order to get the prescription, even threatening to use excessive amounts of alcohol or to commit suicide unless given a prescription.

Demanders are sometimes given benzodiazepines because the doctor hopes to engage them in treatment that will perhaps turn the situation around. My personal experience is that this approach invariably ends in failure, doomed because of the set of false expectations present from the outset. The patient believes that her feelings are unreasonable and can be easily taken away and that the doctor should take them away. If the doctor abets the patient by prescribing benzodiazepines initially, he inadvertently reinforces that patient's beliefs. If the doctor tries at some later point to introduce the idea that learning to tolerate anxiety, rather than just the alleviation of symptoms, is the goal of treatment, the patient can end up feeling betrayed. The inevitable outcome is that the patient continues the drug usage: Either the doctor continues the prescription, or the doctor finally stops prescribing and the patient goes on to find another doctor who will.

Inquirers

Some patients complain of anxiety and are interested in learning about medications. They have no foregone conclusion that medication will be useful for them. Inquirers want to know about the possible benefits, but they also listen if told that these drugs do have some negative side effects and that it is preferable to avoid them because of those side effects. Inquirers are not necessarily seeking a drug at any cost, they want to know both sides of the risk/benefit balance.

Inquirers can often be helped if they are given reassurance by a sympathetic doctor who explains that their symptoms of anxiety are a sign from the body that there is a problem that needs to be addressed. They are often greatly relieved to learn that symptoms of anxiety, though uncomfortable, are entirely normal, and that talking about their distressing situation is the best method for coping. In fact, when these people are given a benzodiazepine they often report using only one or two doses. It is unusual for inquirers to become dependent on them.

Hopers

Hopers fall into a middle ground between the other two types. They generally feel unable to manage their distress and may be used to seeking external aids to help them with their feelings. This group is the most receptive to taking a doctor's lead. If the physician thinks that benzodiazepines will take these feelings away, the patient is reinforced in the belief that what he is feeling is unreasonable. The patient is then all too ready to take drugs to deal with his unreasonable feelings. Difficulties arise when these feelings persist, as feelings generally do when a person tries to cover them up. Then the patient and doctor may continue to try to mute the feelings by continuing the pills.

If the doctor instead explains that temporary use of a benzodiazepine can help the patient to function better temporarily, the goal of treatment then becomes quite different. Rather than erasing the feelings that the patient is experiencing, the pills are used to help the patient tolerate them. This allows them to function more effectively for the few days when they feel overwhelmed, but it does not detract from the goal of learning to manage the new situation successfully.

THIRD-PARTY PAYERS

There has been an enormous change in the way medicine is currently being practiced in the United States due to the rising influence of insurance companies and other health care organizations, such as health maintenance organizations (HMOs) or preferred provider organizations (PPOs). A patient and doctor no longer decide together what the appropriate form of treatment is, based on their understanding of the risks and benefits. By and large, these organizations now direct the choice of treatments because they decide which treatments will be paid for.

In order to maximize profits, these organizations cut costs any way they can. The changes resulting from these cost-cutting measures have been devastating to psychiatry. Some of the cost-cutting techniques are common knowledge, but some are hidden in the written agreements that they strike with employers and doctors and thus are not openly acknowledged. Let's look first at those that affect the patient.

Patient

One roadblock is the practice of limiting the choice of physicians. Large HMOs and PPOs do this by requiring doctors to submit their credentials for placement on "panels." They approve only a portion of the applications, claiming this lowers their administrative overhead. However, it also clearly limits a patient's choice of doctors. When the organizations are large, such as Kaiser-Permanente in California, doctors function essentially as employees. In more rural areas, third-party payers compete for patients and doctors. Some HMOs require doctors to sign an exclusive contract with them, meaning that the doctors will not accept payment from other HMOs. The end result of limiting the number of providers that are funded is that a patient's choice is based not on the quality of a provider, or on a recommendation from friends or doctors, but on the few providers that a given company has on a list.

Another common practice used by third-party payers to limit access to treatment is the creation of a "gatekeeper," commonly a primary care provider such as a family practitioner, general practitioner, internist, or pediatrician. The gatekeeper screens all initial problems and permits visits to specialists only for conditions that she can't handle. They must endorse any request for service by another doctor in order for that service to be paid for. This means that if a patient wants to see an orthopedic surgeon for a foot problem or a psychiatrist for anxiety, he must first obtain approval from the gatekeeper. This limits the number of visits to specialists, who tend to charge higher rates than primary care physicians. The fact that primary care physicians often have less training and knowledge about complex medical problems and sometimes provide lower quality care is essentially irrelevant: Cost containment has become the primary goal of providing medical care. The gatekeeper role is of special concern with psychiatric problems, because most primary care providers do not fully understand the range of psychiatric disorders.

Gatekeepers do have the ability to write prescriptions for psychiatric disorders, however, and often do so without performing a comprehensive assessment of what is contributing to a person's distress and designing a treatment plan that would relieve that distress. The *Wall Street Journal* reported on December 1, 1995, in an article subtitled "[Managed Care's] . . . effort to cut costs leads to overuse, misuse of drugs," that eighty percent of antidepressants are now prescribed by primary care physicians.[24]

For example, a colleague of mine saw a patient who was applying to Social Security for disability on the basis of depression that had kept her out of work for more than six months. Her internist had conducted trials of two antidepressants, using inadequate doses for inadequate periods of time. The patient saw a therapist only six times. She was still depressed and unable to work when seen by my colleague. We were both dismayed at the inadequate treatment that this patient had received, which led her to believe that she was helpless and disabled. Standard psychiatric treatment, adequately performed, could have restored her to full employment within a matter of weeks to months. The patient believed that she was incapable of working, all because her doctor and insurance company were concerned about limiting the cost of her care.

Another major way that third-party payers have limited access to appropriate psychiatric treatment is to state that they do not cover long-term problems and they will only pay for a limited number of visits for short-term, focused treatment on a specific problem that is impairing functioning. This is flat-out discrimination against people with psychiatric problems. No other area of medicine has such unfair constraints placed upon a group of patients; people are not denied treatment of hypertension, mild diabetes, ulcers, emphysema, arthritis, or migraine headaches because they are chronic illnesses and often only minimally impair functioning.

Some third-party payers also have "gag orders" forbidding their providers from telling patients of treatment options that are expensive. Doctors have been fired from panels for telling patients that the payer will not provide payment for a treatment that the provider believes is best.

Third-party payers commonly require "preauthorization" of any psychiatric service. This means that a doctor must contact the company after an initial evaluation session, present the case in detail, and hope that the insurance company sees the need for treatment. A subtle technique these companies use to delay this authorization is to have a very small number of people who perform the authorizations. Doctors sometimes wait weeks for a telephone "appointment" to present the case. There is generally a delay before the authorization is granted, which can be enormously troubling to someone who is in significant personal distress.

The authorization process tends to require delicate handling: It is important for a provider to maintain good relations with the third-party payer. I know of one physician who spoke with the reviewer because he felt that the patient, who was suicidal, needed to stay in the hospital more than the three days that the reviewer had authorized. After the argument heated up, the case manager rescinded her previous authorization for three days and stated that *no* treatment would be authorized.

HMOs and PPOs routinely deny requests for long-term therapy because it is seen as too costly. Since they can't make the argument that long-term therapy is ineffective (too many studies have documented its usefulness), they generally authorize four or eight sessions and tell the doctor that authorization must be sought again after those initial sessions have been held. Since long-term therapy depends on regularity, consistency, and patience in order to be effective, no sensible clinician begins it under these conditions. Instead, the focus becomes helping the patient make some short-term adjustment, even if the underlying problem is left untreated and will likely cause problems in the future.

Finally, many of these organizations routinely refuse to pay for psychiatrists to perform psychotherapy at all, because it is cheaper to hire clinicians who have received less training and who will accept lower fees.

Providers

Besides the constraints on patients, there are many limitations on providers as well. Doctors across the country are worried that they will be cut out of panels and lose their practice because they know it *has* happened to many providers. This leads them to be sensitive to the requirements of third-party payers. Unfortunately, the needs of the patient often get lost. For example, providers need to ensure that they do not develop a "bad" profile of providing care for clients—i.e., a profile demonstrating that their treatment recommendations cost more than those suggested by the "average" provider. When you walk into a provider's office, therefore, your needs are measured against the needs of other patients the doctor has seen. If she goes to bat very strongly for you, then somebody else will lose out. If she goes to bat very strongly for everybody, then she may get cut out of the panel and lose her source of income. This leads most doctors to minimize the treatment that they recommend for people.

Although the concept of a gatekeeper may appear to make sense on the surface, most patients are unaware that a gatekeeper's income is partially dependent on the number of outside referrals that he or she makes. If a gatekeeper refers out "too many" people, he will be penalized financially. If a gatekeeper refers out very few people, on the other hand, he will be financially rewarded. This is accomplished by paying the gatekeeper only ninety percent of what they bill, funding the additional ten percent at the end of the year if their profile is advantageous to the company. The end result is that the gatekeeper will be much less likely to refer patients out for care.

Third-party payers also hide behind the "appeal" process. This is triggered when a doctor or patient feels that the third-party payer has not authorized payment for an appropriate level of service. Essentially, the doctor goes over the head of the initial case reviewer for the third party payer in hopes that she can get the decision reversed by a superior. This is time-consuming, obviously, and often ineffective. Meanwhile, the patient continues to be distressed. It is up to the patient and the doctor to decide whether or not to continue treatment while they are waiting for the decision. However, if the choice is to continue treatment, and the third-party payer denies payment, either the patient has to come up with the money himself, or the doctor decides that she will be providing free care. I recently learned of a contract in which the insurance company prohibits a provider from obtaining payment from the patient in the event that the appeal is denied even if the patient is willing to pay. Third-party payers show this provision to employers when they are selling their policies and communicate to the employers that employees may be able to get free care through this policy. It doesn't take a genius to realize that doctors cannot go through this regularly with all their patients and be caught in the position of providing enormous amounts of free care. The result, of course, is that doctors tend not to appeal.

All of these cost-cutting techniques are enormously profitable for these organizations, as the million-dollar bonuses to their executives make clear, and has resulted in marked limitations of psychiatric services, especially for long-term therapy. So when you come in with anxiety that is intense, unpleasant, and making it hard for you to function, what is a doctor to recommend? Even when doctors are knowledgeable about treatments other than drugs, they know that treatments designed to help a patient understand the causes of anxiety are unlikely to be approved. In writing a prescription, they can provide at least partial help. The end result of the limitations caused by the unwillingness of third-party payers to fund appropriate treatment is that many patients and doctors use benzodiazepines for quick relief of anxiety and ignore the underlying causes.

The limitations on appropriate psychiatric care in HMOs were documented in a review of mental health services provided to 9000 people treated for medical problems in six HMOs across the country and presented in 1997.[25] More than 75 percent of those on psychiatric medications had no psychiatric diagnosis documented in the chart. Less than 10 percent of elderly patients who had a psychiatric diagnosis or were given medication ever saw a mental health specialist, and of those who did, the majority were seen for only one or two visits. A prescription for a benzodiazepine was the most common medication for the treatment of the elderly with depression. Anti-anxiety agents, predominantly benzodiazepines, were the sole psychopharmacological treatment for 16 percent of the elderly with a documented diagnosis of depression.

As we have seen, many forces influence the roles of all five participants who combine to create the Benzo Blues. Underlying all of them is a current that runs deeply through our society and much of mankind: our wish to avoid and ignore any sign of mental weakness. While most of us believe that people should seek treatment for a physical disorder such as cancer, AIDS, or heart disease, even if the treatment is useless for many of them, we believe that people with psychiatric problems should get by with the absolute minimum help. This pervasive stigma against mental illness manifests itself throughout the health care system and plays a role in the inadequate psychiatric treatment that many people receive.

Thus, while even a minor alteration in physical health typically leads many people to call their primary care doctor, patients are embarrassed to have psychiatric problems and often avoid facing any psychiatric distress until they are so troubled that they think they might have a nervous breakdown. They are often ashamed of and hide any psychiatric treatment that they do receive. Doctors fall prey to stigma too, often feeling uncomfortable telling patients that their problems are "all in the head" and focusing their efforts only on the physical aspects of a person's illness. Ignoring the significant component played by a person's psychological state, they order expensive time-consuming tests for symptoms that are clearly due to stress, not any physical illness. Third-party payers openly discriminate against people with mental illness by establishing arbitrary limits on coverage of psychiatric disorders, a practice that does not occur with physical illnesses. Pharmaceutical companies prey on people's shame about psychological problems and tout drugs as a painless solution. And, of course, the popularity of benzodiazepines is due to their wonderful ability to cover up uncomfortable feelings about difficult and painful subjects.

These forces can be very powerful, acting together to persuade a person to ignore the distress inside them. They shape the response of both patient and doctor alike toward what appears to be an easy solution—the prescription and consumption of benzodiazepines. As millions of people have found, however, this easy answer turns out to be no solution but, instead, the beginning of a long road that only goes downhill.

Recent work on anxiety and people with anxiety disorders delineates more specifically how the process of pathological anxiety unfolds. In the next chapter we will look at how and why the patients described earlier became vulnerable to developing an anxiety disorder. This will give us a deeper understanding of how people become dependent on benzos, and also point the way for them to master their anxiety, get off benzodiazepines, and move on in their lives.

· 5 ·

TRAUMA AND THE PROCESS OF PATHOLOGICAL ANXIETY

Pathological anxiety often appears on the surface to be an excessive or inappropriate reaction to current issues in a person's life. For example, Susan felt anxious when her relationship with a boyfriend became more serious, Marilyn continued to feel anxious long after her husband died, and Jim became anxious when his wife became pregnant. But this raises an important question: Why do some people, but not others, have such an excessive reaction to current life events?

It is believed by many that people with pathological anxiety are no different from anyone else and that they weren't anxious at all until the onset of their "pathological" anxiety. However, if one investigates all areas of a person's life, paying special attention to how a person has experienced and handled anxiety in the past, one learns that this is not the case. With systematic questioning, eighty percent of people with panic attacks who were initially unable to say what it was that caused their symptoms were able to identify one or more negative life events preceding their first panic attack. These events include the death of a friend, marital conflict, major surgery, and stress at work.[1] Other authors have also documented that traumatic experiences lead to an increased rate of anxiety disorders.[2] My own clinical experience supports this finding. Often this exploration requires at least some weeks or months of psychotherapy.

Why do some people experience pathological anxiety at all? What makes them different from people who don't? Although Betsy and Sam did not have any apparent difficulties prior to their traumas, their subsequent development of anxiety as part of PTSD can give us some clues about how chronic anxiety develops in people without obvious trauma.

Betsy, the teacher who survived a classroom fire, never discussed her experience with anyone; she just tried to "get over it" by ignoring it and relying on Klonopin. Sam the Vietnam veteran, had a more complex experience. He commented, "I was young going into the service—I was only eighteen. I thought I could handle anything when I was on my way over. But it was more intense than anything I'd imagined." He felt that he'd received no help from the military to put his experience into some kind of perspective and that, as a soldier, he was actively disliked by the American public. Further, one of the peculiarities of the Vietnam War was that soldiers were not sent in tight-knit groups but instead were rotated into units one by one. This had the effect of leaving each soldier virtually on his own emotionally because he joined a unit in Vietnam in which he knew no one.

The fact that Sam and Betsy received no help in processing their feelings and coming to some satisfactory resolution about them led them to hold on to these feelings, which continued to affect them. We know from veterans of many wars and from women who have been raped as adults that development of subsequent psychological distress is less likely if they discuss with other people their thoughts and feelings about what happened. Family and friends can be of significant help with this, but often people need to speak with professionals who are knowledgeable about the complex feelings that arise from trauma. The sooner the person reviews the experience and puts it into some kind of perspective, the better.

So what is the connection to people who experience pathological anxiety without suffering any obvious trauma as adults? If we question anxious people about events in their lives, we find that they have experienced trauma; it just wasn't recent. They experienced trauma earlier in their lives, when they were children.

The connections between early trauma and current anxiety are often unclear initially, but there is a general process that unfolds in people who have experienced childhood trauma. This process leads to lifelong difficulties, one of which is the vulnerability to the lure of benzodiazepines. I will outline this process in some detail because this will further our understanding of why some people develop the Benzo Blues, and how to help them get out of it.

CHILDHOOD TRAUMA

Any child's ability to cope with the experiences of life has limitations. If a particular experience exceeds those limitations, the child will be overwhelmed with a number of feelings, including anxiety, and these feelings will last long after the trauma is over. If children are able to sort out what they are feeling and to take some steps to rebound from the trauma, then the long-term effects are significantly lessened. This always requires the aid of parents and/or other adults. The intensity of the feelings will remain, however, if the child is not helped to rebound. Then the process of becoming a victim of anxiety will begin.

As an aid in seeing the process common to all traumas that leads to chronic anxiety, let's look at some of the different types of trauma that can lead children to experience chronic anxiety.

Early Parental Death

Parental loss prior to the age of eighteen leads to an increased risk of developing panic disorder and different phobias as adults.[3] How does this happen? We recall that Marilyn appeared to become anxious only after her husband died, apparently because of new responsibilities that overwhelmed her. In reality, however, she had never learned how to make independent decisions for herself. She had grown up in a home in which her father made the decisions. As a child, Marilyn saw her mother accept a dependent role because of feelings of inadequacy. But Marilyn's mother had always been aware that she felt stifled and didn't want Marilyn to repeat her mistakes. She encouraged Marilyn to become independent. She arranged for her to learn to ride a horse. She regularly took her to the town library and encouraged her to read widely. Mother and daughter talked a lot about their hope that Marilyn would be able to attend college so that she would have wider options as an adult.

After her mother died, Marilyn was anxious and uncertain about how to negotiate the world successfully. She missed her mother's support and encouragement. She especially missed the day-to-day discussions of her hopes and dreams about different parts of her life. Her mother was wonderful at asking questions that helped Marilyn figure out what she thought, felt, and wanted. Her father meant well, but his way of helping was to give advice rather than helping her discover what she wanted to do, and his recommendations were based on his own values and beliefs, not Marilyn's own wishes and hopes. This pattern of advice giving led Marilyn to feel even more anxious because she felt that she never knew how to make decisions in accordance with her own feelings.

Marilyn grew to mistrust her ability to make her own decisions and increasingly relied instead on her father. She managed the anxiety that people naturally feel when they start making important decisions for themselves by saying to herself, "I might be wrong. My father is older and has more experience; I'd better go along with what he says." In the years after her mother's death, Marilyn became even more uncertain about what she felt and wanted and more helpless when faced with decisions. For example, she wanted to go to college after high school. Her father, however, told her that a college education was useless for a woman. Rather than trying to finance college, she should make use of her typing skills as a secretary. Marilyn followed his advice. Her father's suggestion may have made sense in the short run—college was expensive; working brought in income—but the messages behind it were that she should value money more than her own desires, that she was impractical, that she didn't know what was best for her, and that she wasn't worth educating at a higher level. What's more, this was only one of many times that Marilyn's father had told her what to do, and she complied.

Because Marilyn almost never made significant decisions for herself, she neither experienced successes nor learned from mistakes. Specifically, she developed little sense of herself as someone who could manage reasonable financial decisions. The pattern continued after her marriage. Each time there was a decision to make about money, Marilyn, unsure what to do, would feel a little anxious and then defer to her husband's judgment. Over a twenty-five-year period these sorts of decisions naturally occurred frequently, and included major things like buying cars, purchasing a house, saving for retirement and for the children's college education, and determining how much life insurance to carry. Marilyn also deferred to her husband's wishes on smaller decisions, such as vacation plans. The outcome of the decisions her husband made is not the point here—in fact, Marilyn was rather happy with them—but rather that she continued to feel unable to make decisions herself.

This feeling of inadequacy was reinforced each time the need for a decision arose. Though she was somewhat unaware of it, she had developed the belief that she was a weak and ineffective person who was incapable of making decisions. She felt inadequate about her abilities in many areas of her life, though her doubts about her ability to make financial decisions were the most acute following her husband's death.

When her husband died, therefore, Marilyn had to deal not only with the terrible grief of losing her spouse, but also with the fact that she could no longer rely on her husband to make decisions for her. Most other people who lose a spouse after many years experience significant grief but are not paralyzed by anxiety as they face life as a single person. This is because they have not ceded to their spouse functions that they felt too anxious to perform themselves. As a widow Marilyn would have to make decisions on her own—something that she had never done. It was at this point that her anxiety became so intense that it was "pathological."

Jim also developed anxiety as an adult for no apparent reason. As he himself noted, he should have been happy that his wife was pregnant. He gave the clue to what had been traumatic for him in his first session with me, though. He said, "I always said I'd never let my kids down the way my father let me down. He died when I was only eight." In future sessions, he went on to relate that he had vowed when his father died to be "strong" and not show any "childish" emotions. He refused to cry. His mother would be able to depend on him—he wouldn't let her down. And in fact, he didn't let her down. He studied hard in school and worked part-time to contribute to the family income. But the veneer of self-sufficiency covered up a strong fear that he wouldn't be able to do everything that he "should." This concern is normal in an eight-year-old boy and usually recedes gradually as age-appropriate real life achievements occur. Jim never had a chance to work this concern through gradually, however, because his father's untimely death led him to attempt it all at once. This veneer also covered up his anger at losing his father and at losing the opportunity to do the more playful things that he saw his friends do.

Jim was able to "be strong," but only by single-mindedly focusing on what he "should" do, and by cutting off his sadness, playfulness, and longing for closeness and tenderness. As a person grows through the teenage years and into adulthood, these feelings are normally expressed in different ways, allowing him to learn new ways of interacting with other people. For example, a close same-sex chum in elementary school can help a child learn a lot about how to relate in intimate relationships with either sex in later years. But Jim didn't share his feelings with others, and these emotions didn't have a chance to mature. The result was that he was virtually incapable of dropping his "strong" veneer even to play with his new baby daughter. The diminished feelings that his coping style allowed and what he knew good fathers "should" be like produced a true conflict that couldn't be resolved without something changing. This conflict led Jim to experience intense anxiety as an adult—but the conflict and the anxiety over what he "should" do and what he really wanted to do had been inside him since his father's death.

Marilyn and Jim reacted very differently to the death of a parent when they were children due in part to their family dynamics, their sex, and their own personalities. But each experienced tremendous feelings of helplessness and anxiety. Although they reacted very differently, they both carried the anxiety inside them for many years until they faced situations as an adult that forced them to confront their earlier feelings and the coping styles that had now proven ineffective.

Sexual Abuse

Though Heather, the young lawyer with "unspecified anxiety," didn't dwell on her experiences with her father in recounting her history to me, I knew full well the devastating impact that sexual abuse has on the development of a person's sense of self and the struggle to find a sense of safety in the world.

In the eighties and nineties many people became aware that sexual abuse, previously thought to be quite rare, was, in fact, common. It is difficult to estimate the frequency of sexual abuse both because it is often covered up and because the severity of abuse can be so varied. A landmark study of over nine hundred women found that, by a conservative estimate, some thirty-eight percent of women are sexually abused before the age of eighteen, and twenty-eight percent before the age of fourteen. Some sixteen percent are sexually abused by a relative (i.e., incest) before the age of eighteen.[4] The tremendous outpouring of reports in the media and the scientific literature has shown that sexual abuse causes profoundly negative and long-lasting effects. Adults who have been sexually abused as children have a higher rate of anxiety disorders, depression, and physical complaints.[5] How can the sexual abuse of children lead to anxiety in adults? To answer that question, it is important to understand the childhood experience of sexual abuse.

In her book *Father's Days*, Katherine Brady offers a powerful description of being sexually abused.[6] She presents eloquent and excruciating testimony to the way her father's persistent sexual abuse invaded every aspect of her life, including her relationships with family members and friends, her ability to perform in school, her sense of herself as a person, and the development of her sexual life. Although her surface personality appeared friendly and normal, privately she was fearful, depressed, and anxious.

Brady focuses on two aspects of her life that led her to be chronically anxious. First, she had to be on guard against her father's advances at all times. She tried to avoid being alone with her father because he persistently forced her to have sex. She was most fearful on Saturday mornings because that was when her mother generally ran her errands. She usually asked her mother not to go, or asked to go along. She used any argument to try to convince her father not to abuse her. She tried to avoid being alone with him on camping trips or vacations, attempting to be otherwise occupied or in the midst of other people so that she wouldn't be alone with him.

A second source of Brady's anxiety was the fear that other people might learn her secret. Her father warned her not to tell her mother because she would become angry. Petrified that she and her father would be discovered, she asked him to institute a family rule that the house should be locked at all times. She was also afraid that her mother, smelling the odor they left or seeing the towels he used, would suspect what was happening. Never close to her somewhat cold and distant mother, Brady quickly realized that her mother didn't want to know what was happening; she wanted to preserve the illusion of a happy family and didn't want to jeopardize the marriage. Thus, Brady was forced into a life of secrecy. As she grew up, Brady's chronic feelings of anxiety persistently and continuously shaped her behavior in destructive ways. She developed dependent relationships with other people rather than relating as equals. Rather than developing a career for herself, she sought a boyfriend to marry in the hope that he would take care of her financially. As she aged she continued to feel anxious.

Many adults who were sexually abused as children continue to suffer from overwhelming symptoms of anxiety. They are anxious for many of the same reasons that Brady is. They are anxious that someone will find out their secret. They are anxious that someone will hurt them again if they get too close. They are anxious that people they meet will think they are bad. They often try to forget the experience and are anxious anytime something reminds them of it. Some are unaware that they are anxious because they are able to keep it under wraps, but many are aware of the ongoing battle against feeling too anxious. Many have panic attacks. Some have PTSD. This can make them an easy target for drugs, like benzodiazepines, that seem to offer relief and support in the daily struggle against feeling overwhelmed.

Parental Alcohol Abuse

Sometimes a person's "trauma" has not as obvious a cause as war, parental death, or sexual abuse. For example, Debbie experienced agoraphobia only as an adult, but she had experienced significant anxiety very early in her life. Although her anxiety possibly had a genetic/biological component, it was worsened by her father's drinking. On a superficial level, his behavior while drinking intensified her shyness to the point that she didn't invite friends over to her house. More important, though, her shyness was ignored because her parents were preoccupied with drinking.

The growth of Alcoholics Anonymous, as well as offshoots such as Adult Children of Alcoholics, has contributed greatly to our understanding of how devastating this experience can be. Numerous books and articles describe the many facets of this complex trauma. What occurs, however, is very simple. The child's needs are neglected because of the parent's continued use of alcohol. As Wayne Kritsberg has pointed out in *The Adult Children of Alcoholics Syndrome,* alcoholic parents do not supply their children with consistent love and support.[7] This neglect can result in both physical and emotional abandonment. Physical abandonment can take the form of missed meals, being left alone for hours, or being left in the care of older siblings who are still children themselves.

Although many children with alcoholic parents have their basic physical needs met, Kritsberg feels that they are all emotionally abandoned to some degree, in part because the parents are drinking and don't focus on the child's feelings. The distress they feel also occurs because their parents clearly manage their own distress inadequately (that's why they drink) and so cannot help a child learn appropriate ways to overcome difficulties.

According to Kritsberg, children of alcoholic parents feel many overwhelming emotions—including fear, anger, hurt, resentment, distrust, loneliness, and sadness—because of the emotional abandonment. Kritsberg feels that primary among these feelings is the fear that they will not survive and that their emotions will bubble up from the inside and overwhelm them. They often experience chronic anxiety.[8] Female children of alcoholics may be especially vulnerable. They have a lower sense of self-esteem and more anxiety than do men.[9]

Many children of alcoholics manage these feelings by restricting both feelings and behavior and assuming a narrow, tightly defined role within the family. This allows children to feel that there is some order and predictability in their lives in spite of the manifest chaos and their intense feelings. Kritsberg describes the roles of the enabler, who helps protect the alcoholic from experiencing the consequences of his behavior; the placater, who tries to lessen tension in the family by trying to smooth things over and avoiding any direct expression of feelings or wishes; and the clown, who lessens tension in the family by being funny and cute. The "responsible" one is the child who assumes an inordinate share of responsibility for her own behavior and for others.[10] The "lost" child never asserts his own needs within the family, in part because no one is listening. There are many other roles. No person fits neatly into one role, and the roles may shift from person to person as the family changes over time.

Although these roles allow children to find an outlet for some of their feelings, others remain inside unexpressed. It can be difficult for them to break out of their roles in other situations. For example, when enablers develop their own relationships as adults, they tend to focus on meeting the needs of the other person and ignore their own needs. They may be quite clear about what they want emotionally from others but are unable to obtain it. Everyone likes the placater, but no one, including the placater himself, knows what he wants. The clown can be funny but may find it difficult to persist in any endeavor, such as school, that requires serious effort for an extended period of time. The responsible one must always be in control of a situation and doesn't know how to relax and enjoy life. The lost child often seeks out involvement with groups during adolescence and adulthood that provide a source of identity, such as religious organizations. As the child of an alcoholic grows into adulthood, these characteristic styles of living become ingrained and then strangling.

These ingrained roles may be marginally successful in helping a child survive a painful childhood, but can be disastrous in adult life for the simple reason that the challenges of life as an adult are quite different from those of childhood. For example, placaters "typically go through years of adulthood never seriously considering what they want, rather, they are forever discounting their needs. They have trained themselves to be only concerned with providing for others. The consequence of this behavior is that they never get what they want." Chris, a "responsible" child, "had so organized and structured her own childhood, she became a very rigid person, lacking in flexibility. As a child, Chris needed to be in charge, or at least feel that she was in control; if she was not, she had a sense that her entire world was collapsing around her. For Chris, the adult, this phenomenon continues. She finds herself needing to take charge, to feel in absolute control, or there is a pervading sense of losing control and being totally overwhelmed." Joe, another "responsible" child, felt that the loss of control was intolerable. These people are building their whole lives around being "in control" and avoiding the anxiety that the loss of control would cause.[11]

As we have seen, Debbie, the young woman with agoraphobia, minimized her contact with the outside world as a child in order to minimize her anxiety about her parents' drinking and her own ability to negotiate the tasks of the world successfully. She was "lost," without a clear idea of what she wanted and how she would obtain it. As an adult, she still lived at home, and she worked for a boss who offered to help her get ahead with some health benefits and further education. But when she learned that she might have cancer, her unconscious fear that the world was *never* going to be safe for her seemed to become a reality. This blunted any relief that the normal results of the follow-up Pap smear would usually give somebody. She continued taking the Librium but never learned how to manage her anxiety any other way, and was unable to take charge of herself and her life.

Divorce

Another long-lasting experience that is traumatic for many children is parental divorce. For instance, when she first came in, Susan denied that she had feelings about her parents' divorce, but she did acknowledge that this experience made her extremely wary of getting close in a romantic relationship. Her initial experience with panic attacks came during a time of increasing closeness in her first serious relationship.

Judith Wallerstein, Ph.D., is the founder and executive director of the Center for the Family in Transition, located in California, and has followed a sizable number of families as they have gone through the process of divorce and its aftermath. In her first book, *Surviving the Breakup* (1980), Wallerstein described how each person in the family reacts to a divorce. She focused especially on the difficulties of children, describing a number of emotional responses that were common to all of them. Divorce is frightening for children because the assurance of continued nurturance and protection, which has been implicit in an intact family, no longer exists. They had many worries, some realistic, some less so, but "the anxiety itself was a widespread phenomenon, and appeared as a central response."[12]

The children worried about who would take care of them, who would feed them, who would protect them, or whether they would be placed in foster homes. Half were afraid of abandonment by their father and one-third by their mother. Eighteen months after the divorce, twenty percent of the children evaluated still experienced anxiety. A quarter continued to be intensely unhappy. Five years after the divorce, thirty-seven percent had become depressed. Some of the depressed children also continued to experience anxiety.

In *Second Chances* (1989), Wallerstein followed up on the children she had interviewed earlier as they reached their twenties and found that even children who did well in high school and who had many friends and stable relationships experienced rising anxiety in their late teens and early twenties. She also described the "sleeper effect," in which girls who were previously felt to be functioning well had difficulty establishing a romantic relationship. "A significant number of young women are living with an intolerable level of anxiety about betrayal. So preoccupied are they with expectations of betrayal that they really suffer minute to minute, even though their partners may be completely faithful. Girls who have never been betrayed by either parent fear betrayal. Girls who have never been betrayed or abandoned by a lover fear betrayal and abandonment."[13]

Wallerstein's work presented many new findings about the effects of divorce on children's lives. Her studies clearly demonstrate that many children feel intense anxiety at the time of the divorce and for decades afterward. She estimates that each year between 1972 and 1979 a million new children under eighteen experienced the divorce of their parents. This means that millions and millions of children are growing up feeling intense anxiety. Many will also experience it as adults.

Susan may have felt that her panic attacks came out of the blue, but in fact her parents' separations and divorce had left her feeling chronically anxious. She stayed on Ativan to manage her panic attacks and her anticipatory anxiety but was unaware of the underlying cause of her anxiety.

Other Traumas

Physical abuse, poverty, natural disasters, a significant absence of a parent due to physical illness, and the emotional neglect that can occur with parents who have depression or other forms of mental illness can also profoundly shape children's experience. Trauma can come in many forms. Tom's experience of social phobia helps us to understand this.

Tom did not appear to experience any major trauma when he grew up. His parents stayed together, didn't drink, and didn't abuse him physically. But Tom's social phobia led him to become a target of emotional abuse by his father. His incessant teasing, public humiliation, and constant communication that he wasn't good enough and needed to be "toughened up" all left their mark. Although his father may have meant well, his constant harassment led Tom to become even more sensitive and worried about how others perceived him and even more insecure about his own abilities. In fact, Tom needed the opposite approach during his childhood—some recognition that he was uncomfortable with others and a great deal of support in learning ways to overcome his fearfulness. For instance, his father might have encouraged him to take a public speaking course to help practice feeling comfortable in front of an audience, or his father might have helped him to learn some wilderness survival skills through camping and canoeing so that Tom would feel more confident of his own abilities.

As an adult Tom continued to be insecure about his abilities and anxious that anyone would think he was inadequate. His main coping style was either to avoid uncomfortable situations or ignore his anxiety and just force himself to go ahead. When he chanced upon a boss who shared some of his father's intrusive and critical qualities, he became even more anxious, and his previous coping strategies became ineffective. It was at this point that he sought relief from the Tranxene.

Janet, the seventy-five-year-old woman with health problems, didn't appear to have any dramatic traumatic experiences growing up either. In fact, she always told herself that she had had a good life early on. In doing so, however, she had to minimize the emotional deprivations that occurred because her mother had to go to work outside the home, leaving Janet to assume the role of a parent at age eleven. She organized her siblings to help with the laundry but had to prod them to get it done. She had to buy food with very little money and prepare meals. She had to manage the day-to-day problems of her siblings, like sickness, even though she was still a child herself. At times she was intensely anxious because she feared that she wouldn't be able to accomplish everything. Further, the concrete details of her life were so consuming that she ignored her own feelings of sadness and anger at her lot. She just knew that she had to put aside her own hopes, and she wasn't able to continue her education because she always had to be at home to care for her younger siblings.

As she reached her twenties, Janet's siblings continued to need help, and to help them she continued to repress her own dreams. She wanted to have children of her own, but there never seemed to be time to go out with men. After one brother lost an arm in World War II, he needed help dressing, bathing, shopping, and learning how to get around. A younger sister developed tuberculosis, and after two years in a sanitarium, she returned home "cured" but in need of help to get back on her feet. As her siblings got married and started their families, Janet fell into the role of baby-sitter and family organizer. She kept helping, but her feelings of sadness and anger remained inside her. She bottled them up, but in so doing, she also bottled up her hopes to establish her own life. She had many different medical problems including painful menstruation, an irritable bowel with nausea and diarrhea, and bouts of light-headedness. She frequently saw doctors because the symptoms would often overwhelm her, but no major problems were ever found.

Finally, when she went through menopause, Janet realized that she never would have her own family. She bottled up this realization and the feelings associated with it as well, however, in what was now a long-standing pattern. She was intermittently anxious and sad but would shrug off the distressing feelings by insisting that she was just feeling sorry for herself. It was at this time that her colitis worsened. She had always appreciated the attention she received from members of the medical profession, an experience that was unusual in her life. It was their job, and she wasn't burdening them as she would if she expressed her concerns to her family, and as she herself had been burdened by her family's needs. She first received prescriptions for Serax during this period to help her through times when she was anxious.

When she developed hypertension, however, she realized that she wasn't as invulnerable as she had always thought. She might have a stroke and need people to take care of her. The thought that she might need to depend on others shook her sense of identity as a strong, independent person to the core. She became anxious and couldn't shrug it off. Even with the Serax she couldn't relax. She developed headaches and began taking Fiorinal. She took Restoril to sleep. Her colitis flare-ups grew more frequent and more severe. Her requests for medical attention to Dr. Crandal and his staff grew more frequent.

Although Dr. Crandal thought he was doing the best that he could for Janet by tending conscientiously to her medical needs, both he and Janet avoided any significant discussion of what was really making her anxious. Although the Serax calmed her, however, taking it aided the avoidance. As a result, Janet's anxiety continued unaddressed for years and worsened as the medical problems of old age began to accumulate.

MITIGATING FACTORS

Why do "only" a few million people become dependent on benzo-diazepines when many tens of millions of people experience trauma? I chose to describe the traumatic experiences in the first part of this chapter because most people can intuitively see that they would cause distress and anxiety in children. It is not such a great leap to see that these events might lead people to be anxious as adults. But children who are traumatized can have very different experiences, depending on what else is happening in their lives at the time of the trauma and afterward. These mitigating factors can shape the experience of trauma in myriad ways.

The degree and type of damage resulting from traumatic experiences can vary tremendously depending on the type of trauma, its severity, and the degree of intrusiveness to an individual.[14] A girl whose brother touches her inappropriately two or three times when she is thirteen has a very different experience from that of a girl whose father engages her in intercourse from the age of five to fifteen. Likewise, parents who divorce and try to keep a strong focus on the needs of the children as the divorce proceeds create a very different experience for their children than parents who use their children as weapons in their postmarital war. A father who drinks regularly on nights and weekends but who is otherwise a reasonable parent creates a very different atmosphere than a father who is frequently absent and becomes physically abusive when drinking.

The child can bring different qualities to a situation, too. For example, a child who is smart, good-looking, and athletically gifted may be able to develop outside relationships that can lessen the impact of the trauma. By contrast, children who do poorly in school and who don't make friends easily may alienate potential sources of support. This may lead them to have a difficult time at school as well as at home, so there is no arena in which they feel good about their life.

In addition, other people's positive involvement can substantially shape the experience of a child who has been traumatized. Teachers, adult friends, and relatives can be very important in helping a child to develop in positive ways even when the trauma continues. Good psychiatric treatment at almost any age can also be enormously beneficial to people who have been traumatized in order to help them to put the trauma in perspective and to manage the remaining effects as well as possible.

The importance of childhood trauma to the development of pathological anxiety has been minimized in the last fifteen years or so with the rise of the "biological revolution." This has had many unfortunate effects, one of which is the tendency for doctors and patients alike to use benzodiazepines to cover up feelings rather than to employ psychotherapy and other forms of treatment to uncover and resolve them more satisfactorily. Once begun, the strategy of relying on drugs merely continues the unsuccessful efforts used by people to block out painful feelings from trauma, and interferes with the process of correcting the root of anxiety.

Up until now we have focused on the similarities in the lives of people with the Benzo Blues. Chapter 6, however, will focus on understanding a major difference: why women have a higher rate of dependency than men.

◆ 6 ◆

WOMEN, MEN, ANXIETY, AND BENZOS

When Susan experienced her first panic attack, with symptoms of chest pain, palpitations, and difficulty breathing, she was terrified and went to the emergency room. She was relieved when the physician there assured her that she was not having a heart attack but a panic attack, and gave her a shot of Ativan for her symptoms. She felt better within the hour. The psychiatrist that Susan consulted at the advice of the ER doctor agreed that she should continue with the Ativan.

A prescription is influenced by many more factors than merely a person's symptoms of anxiety. Because Susan's experience is so common, even those who are somewhat leery of the use of benzodiazepines might miss a very salient point: The patient is a woman. As numerous studies have documented, women are given prescriptions for benzodiazepines twice as frequently as men.[1]

Besides taking these drugs more frequently, women also experience anxiety disorders more frequently than men.[2] Although a number of clinicians had documented this for many years in small samples, it was confirmed when the U.S. Government National Institute of Mental Health surveyed more than twenty thousand adults between the ages of eighteen and fifty-four.[3] Women experience social phobia forty percent more often, and panic disorder 150 percent more often. Overall, women experience anxiety disorders sixty percent more frequently than men.

There are two separate issues that these numbers raise. First, why do women experience anxiety disorders more frequently? Second, it appears that benzodiazepines are prescribed disproportionately to women. The prescription rate is 2:1, yet the rate of anxiety disorders in women is only about 1.6:1. What is the reason for this disproportionate prescribing?

An explanation of both disparities can be found by examining four issues: the differences in the way that men and women experience anxiety; the differences in the way that they seek help for their anxiety from the medical profession; the different ways that they are viewed and treated by the medical profession; and the different motivations that lead them to take medication once prescribed.

DO WOMEN AND MEN EXPERIENCE ANXIETY DIFFERENTLY?

As we saw earlier, anxiety disorders are best understood by examining three realms of a person's life: the biological, the social, the psychological. Is there any evidence that women differ from men in these three realms, which might influence their experience of anxiety?

Biological

As we saw in chapter 4, the anatomical apparatus that produces the outward manifestations of anxiety appears identical in women and men. Jerome Kagan, an observer of infant behavior and author of *The Nature of the Child,* notes a wide variation in infants' expression of anxiety, but no inherent differences in the range of expression on the basis of sex.[4] Mary Ainsworth, an observer and researcher of children for decades and the author of *Patterns of Attachment,* pioneered the "Strange Situation" experimental paradigm to study the quality of attachment in hundreds of infants and children.[5] This "Strange Situation" research observes the child's reaction when briefly left alone with a stranger and when the mother returns. In concordance with Kagan, Ainsworth found no apparent difference between the sexes in their demonstration of anxiety toward strangers in the first year of life.

It is possible that there are biological factors that manifest themselves later in life. For example, males and females are subject to different levels of sexual hormones such as testosterone, estrogen, and progesterone during and after puberty, and these hormones might affect the neurological apparatus differently. Many women experience increased anxiety and depression as the progesterone falls toward the end of the second half of the menstrual cycle, commonly referred to as premenstrual syndrome, or PMS. There is little research, however, evaluating the presence of anxiety disorders during other periods of hormonal shifts such as pregnancy and menopause. Although many women and clinicians note an increase in the level of anxiety during menopause, many other factors besides hormonal shifts contribute to this increase, including feelings about aging and childbearing. There is as yet no accepted understanding of how stress, the menstrual cycle, and anxiety can affect each other. Overall then, there is no specific evidence linking hormonal differences to a higher rate of anxiety disorders in women.

Social

Victimization by external trauma is one root cause of anxiety and anxiety disorders. Is it possible that women have an experience of trauma different from men?

One difference is that women are the victims of physical trauma more frequently than men. They have smaller physiques and are made aware at an early age that they need to avoid situations of physical danger. As we saw in the case of Heather, women are victims of sexual abuse as girls and rape as adults far more often than men. They are more likely to be the victim of spouse abuse. Finally, they are more frequently dependent financially so that, as Marilyn found, disruptions in family life can be anxiety provoking for realistic financial as well as emotional reasons.

Although the higher frequency of trauma to women certainly contributes to their higher frequency of anxiety disorders, it cannot, by itself, account for the differential effects. Women are more likely than men to develop an anxiety disorder such as PTSD or GAD after a disaster that affects both sexes equally, such as the Mount Saint Helens explosion or the Exxon *Valdez* oil spill.[6] Urban women aged twenty-one to thirty were more likely than men to develop PTSD when they witnessed violent events occurring to others.[7]

Psychological

Does some aspect of women's psychology lead to greater vulnerability to anxiety when stressed? Questions like this have sometimes been answered in a cavalier manner that tells more about the assumptions of the person providing the answer than about women. For example, the sexist notion that women are the "weaker sex" still finds supporters. And it is true that our society finds the expression of emotion more tolerable in women than men—it is acceptable for a woman to cry in public, for instance, but men are supposed to keep a stiff upper lip. Thankfully, there are some sensible insights into the psychology of women that can shed some light on this subject.

To locate reasonable challenges to the "weaker sex" point of view, we need to look back to the sixties, when the feminist movement that had been latent in this country since the early part of the century began to gain significant ground. This was a time when many disenfranchised groups, including blacks and Native Americans, began to emerge from powerlessness. Women began to enter a variety of professions that had been previously closed to them such as medicine, psychiatry, and related disciplines in psychology. Their insights into the psychology of women have been quite different from men's.

Women psychologists and psychiatrists such as Judith Herman, author of *Father-Daughter Incest*,[8] Carole Gilligan, author of *In a Different Voice*,[9] and Jean Baker Miller, author of *Toward a New Psychology of Women*,[10] have opened new horizons in our understanding of how men and women experience the world in different ways. *Women's Growth and Connection* (1991) is a landmark book written by five women theorists collaborating at the Stone Center at Wellesley College that changed the way many psychiatrists understand the psychology of women. In the preface, the authors stated "We were troubled . . . by the more pervasive and insidious application to women of models of development inspired by a male culture; these theories consistently mislabeled women as deficient. Thus theories of 'human development' which espoused increasing capacity for separation, autonomy, mastery, independence, and self-sufficiency as indications of health and maturity consistently portrayed women as too emotional, too dependent, lacking clear boundaries, and so forth."[11] Their research into how girls and women think, feel, and act differently from boys and men has led to the development of a new theory of psychology.

Their theory is often termed self-in-relation: "In brief, we are arguing that while existing theories posit some form of autonomy or separation as the developmental path, women's core self-structure, or their primary motivational thrust, concerns growth within relationship, or what we call 'self-in-relation'. . . . What we are emphasizing . . . are the key aspects of attaining a capacity to be attuned to the affect of others, understanding and being understood by the other, and thus participating in the development of others. . . . Connection with others, then, is a key component of action and growth, not a detraction from or a means to one's self-enhancement, as implied in other theories." Through the lens of this theory, the authors have looked at many psychological phenomena, including anger, women's greater tendency toward depression than men, the relationship between mothers and daughters, women and power, and even eating patterns.

What does self-in-relation theory have to say about anxiety? Although women and men alike can experience anxiety for many reasons, self-in-relation theory helps us to understand that women, more so than men, become anxious when an important relationship is jeopardized. For example, Susan's panic attacks had started when she felt dissatisfied in her relationship with Mark many years before. Her anxiety at that time was due to being caught on the horns of a dilemma: whether to tolerate Mark's drinking and domineering behavior and resign herself to periods of loneliness because he would shut her out, or to end the relationship and be alone. No matter which way she turned, she would not be able to achieve and maintain a satisfying and close relationship. With the knowledge gained from the self-in-relation theory, we can see that the idea of disrupting the relationship with Mark went against the core needs of a woman who finds meaning and satisfaction in preserving and enhancing relationships. Susan became anxious, her anxiety was manifested by panic attacks, and she started taking Ativan—as she tried to maintain the relationship with Mark. The relationship eventually broke up anyway. Her anxiety continued, however, because her experience of her parents' fighting, separations, and eventual divorce led her to believe that this conflict would occur no matter who she found.

Some women stay in relationships that are extremely unsatisfactory, even abusive, in order to preserve this sense of connection. Women who stay in an abusive relationship have been negatively characterized as masochistic by some, as if the women were purposely seeking pain. The self-in-relation theory helps us to see that most of these women see themselves as maintaining the relationship in spite of the pain. Such women may seek benzodiazepines to minimize their anxiety about the relationship. At times women have asked me for the drugs because they want something to quiet the constant internal fear that their partners are going to physically harm them.

Although men also have a need for affiliation and connection, they tend to be more focused on their wish for autonomy, mastery, and independence. Elizabeth Ettore, author of *Women and Substance Use* (1994), noted that men tended to become anxious due to concerns about their ability to work.[12] For instance, Jim became anxious when he thought he might not be able to support his children adequately. Since women worry these days about jobs as well, the effect of their self-in-relation anxiety adds an even greater burden.

HOW DO WOMEN AND MEN SEEK HELP FOR ANXIETY?

The two sexes behave differently when they seek help for anxiety and other forms of psychiatric distress. Men are more likely to use alcohol and other substances when stressed, and as a result they have a higher rate of substance abuse disorders than women.[13] They are also more likely to obtain prescription psychiatric drugs for the first time from friends and relatives.[14] Women, on the other hand, are more likely than men to present a medical doctor with physical complaints that have a psychological origin[15] and to seek professional psychiatric help.[16]

The self-in-relation theory helps us to understand this difference. People, primarily men, who value separation, autonomy, independence, and mastery will want to preserve their sense of identity as someone who can "stand alone." They dislike acknowledging any distress, inability to cope, or feelings of vulnerability. This leads them to abuse substances more and to be less likely to seek out a professional with a request for help. They often delay seeking help until they have difficulty functioning at work. Other people, primarily women, who value connection with others and feel that sharing experiences can enhance growth, will actively seek out other people when feeling distressed. They will seek out a professional if their problems are serious or if they are not being heard by people who are important to them. The end result is that more women than men go to a doctor or a psychiatrist when in distress. This likely contributes to their greater use of benzodiazepines.

DO DOCTORS TREAT WOMEN AND MEN DIFFERENTLY?

Three studies suggest that the answer to this question is yes. In one study, women were sixty percent more likely to receive benzodiazepines than men with the same diagnosis.[17] In another, females had more than twice the risk of men of being prescribed psychiatric drugs when they had no diagnosis or a psychiatric diagnosis.[18]

Elizabeth Ettore also addressed this question in her study of one hundred people who had used psychiatric drugs for an average of nine years.[19] About ninety percent took benzodiazepines either alone or in combination with other psychiatric drugs. She states that many patients had grown concerned about the duration of their drug use and asked their doctors to help them stop. Male patients were *twice* as likely to receive support from their doctors in their desire to stop. One-third of women users had been told that there was no alternative to their drug use, while only six percent of men were told this. These studies suggest that the difference in the rate of benzodiazepine prescriptions between women and men does not occur solely because their problems are different but because doctors recommend different treatments for them. None of the studies discuss the treatments that men are offered in place of benzodiazepines.

In *Women and Substance Use*, Ettore states that this is due to society's and the medical profession's interest in maintaining women in a passive and dependent role.[20] Ettore uses the term *passive* to mean not only a lack of physical aggression, but also an acceptance of one's lot in life, even if one is restricted to a confining, subordinate role. She uses the term *dependence* to mean that women depend on others' opinions of them for their own self-worth. To see why she comes to this conclusion, it is useful to look at how the medical profession has treated women in other situations.

First, the field of medicine is part of a larger culture that has discriminated against and oppressed women for centuries. This oppression has taken the form of political marginalization. Women only obtained the ability to vote in this country in the early 1900s, and in many countries they still have no political voice. Financial dependency on men is promoted through suppression of women's endeavors. In the United States women were largely denied admission to institutions such as medical and law schools that offer advanced educational degrees until the sixties, and their attempts to enter the business world were discouraged and even undermined. Also, their experiences have been devalued. Sexual discrimination, abuse, and rape were largely ignored for centuries. Even today, we see how women are devalued in the practice of preferential infanticide of girls in China and India.

Apart from its place in society, the medical profession has always placed a strong emphasis on developing, preserving, and maintaining power over all patients regardless of their needs. For example, organized medicine successfully battled midwives at the turn of the century to take over the practice of obstetrics for itself and continued to discourage the acceptance of non-M.D. specialists, ranging from nurse practitioners to chiropractors. Even now, during the current debate over managed care in this country, the complaint of many doctors is not so much that *patients'* health is impaired by managed care, but that doctors don't have the *autonomy* that they value so highly. Finally, the frequent physician complaint that patients are not "compliant" with their "orders" demonstrates that physicians often see patients as subordinates to be controlled rather than as partners in the shared task of preserving and enhancing health.

Organized medicine has long ignored women's unique medical needs. Many works have documented the many different abuses of women by the medical profession.[21] For example, efforts at finding safe, effective contraception that gives women control over their reproductive health have been blocked by the medical profession for centuries. Women of childbearing age are routinely excluded from major drug studies because their hormonal cycles are considered too complicated to be taken into account. Recent recommendations for women with cardiac problems were actually based on studies that examined only men. Women's health problems such as breast cancer received only minimal funding by the government until the nineties.

Not surprisingly, women's psychological distress has been neglected as well. Although Sigmund Freud was well aware that some women were sexually abused, he chose to formulate his theories and practice as if such abuse did not take place. His theory of female psychology proposed that the cause of women's anxiety and psychological distress was their lack of acceptance of the "feminine role." That is, women should be passive, accepting of their subordinate economic and social status. Unfortunately, generations of psychoanalysts followed Freud's lead, turning their attention away from the victims of sexual abuse and blaming women's distress on their unwillingness to accept their assigned role in life. Psychoanalyst Ralph Greenson, author of the widely influential *The Technique and Practice of Psychoanalysis,* expressed this view succinctly in *Life* magazine in 1955: "Someone has to represent authority, and in our society it should be the male."[22]

Most physicians do not consciously think that they are oppressing women, of course. In fact, women physicians are more likely to prescribe medications to women patients.[23] Nevertheless, women receive psychiatric medications preferentially because of unconscious biases on the part of the medical profession.

DO MOTIVATIONS TO TAKE BENZOS DIFFER BETWEEN MEN AND WOMEN?

Some authors have also understood women's use of benzodiazepines and other tranquilizers as a combination of the wish for control by society and women's own belief that they should be dependent and passive.[24] For example, Ettore states in *Women and Substance Use* that a woman may use benzodiazepines, and other psychotropic drugs, to be consistent with her own desire to be a good girl by being dependent and following the doctor's orders. This desire is due in part to the messages given to young girls that they should be passive and dependent. They are told how to be passive when they hear prohibitions against expressing anger, or criticisms for being aggressive. They are often told, and thus feel, that there is something wrong, something "unladylike," when they experience strong emotions. They are protected more than boys and discouraged from exploring the outside world as early and as fully as boys. All of these can lead girls to develop feelings of dependence and passivity as adults. They may sense that something is wrong and feel inadequate to deal with it but be unsure what it is. When they feel anxious, therefore, they may see themselves as somehow deficient and believe that there is something wrong with them. This need to fix their deficiency may lead them to take a drug that changes them rather than to do something that would change their situation.

Ettore specifically examined the reasons men and women took benzodiazepines.[25] Both survey data and personal interviews suggested that men used drugs because they thought their work was stressful and they needed help. Their use was overt, and the men felt theirs was a legitimate medical need. By contrast, many women used them because of problems with husbands or children. They often felt guilty about their use of drugs, and many tried to keep their use secret from others.

Self-in-relation theory helps us to understand the connection between the feelings of inadequacy and passivity on the one hand, and disruptions in the home that lead women to take benzodiazepines. There are at least four ways benzodiazepines may help a woman preserve her sense of connection.

Benzodiazepines Create Harmony with the World

The main way that benzodiazepines can help someone to feel better is that they mimic good feelings. As with the use of alcohol, they can give people a false sense that things are okay. Michael Balint, an English psychoanalyst, describes this harmony-seeking behavior in alcoholics in *The Basic Fault:* "The first effect of intoxication is invariably the establishment of a feeling that everything is now well between them and their environment. In my experience a yearning for this feeling of 'harmony' is the most important cause of alcoholism or for that matter any form of addiction."[26] Benzodiazepines, sometimes referred to as "freeze-dried martinis," perform the same function.

This false sense of harmony allowed Susan to stay in a relationship with Mark even though she had strong negative feelings about it. Although she preserved the relationship, which was important to her, she suppressed other important feelings. As uncomfortable as these feelings were, they were legitimate and should not have been ignored. And in fact, as Susan experienced, feelings ignored do not go away. They snowball and eventually cause significant distress. Of course, men can experience this false sense of harmony, which can lead them to stay in relationships and situations that are unsatisfying. They also have a need for affiliation and connection, though they may be less aware of it than women. Men, however, are less likely to feel that it is their job to achieve harmony at any price.

Benzodiazepines Provide Connection with Another Person—the Doctor

Most of us have had the experience of taking our troubles to someone in authority. Even without making or experiencing any change in the troubling situation, we often feel better if the person we consult seems to understand how we are feeling. Sharing distress often makes a patient feel less alone and more connected—in this case, to the doctor. This is often the case when a patient sees a physician about a problem and the doctor agrees that he is "certainly having a difficult time." This response validates the person's distress. Practitioners in the mental health field call this feeling of connection the therapeutic "alliance" and know that it can be a powerful aid in helping someone deal with a problem.

If this same doctor prescribes a medication, it can solidify an alliance around the belief that the symptoms are excessive or "wrong." For example, when the psychiatrist Susan consulted described her problem as a "chemical imbalance," she felt as if they were on the same side, fighting an "illness" in her body. He agreed with Susan's assessment that her feelings of anxiety were unreasonable and excessive. His support confirmed her belief that *she* was okay, that it was merely her unruly chemistry that was to blame. In this case, the physician's willingness to prescribe the drug helped to establish a stronger unity between them against her unpleasant feelings of anxiety. Although it was good that the psychiatrist and Susan formed a strong alliance, it was unfortunately used to fight a false enemy. The real problem was not her unruly chemistry, but her unwillingness to learn how to manage the symptoms of anxiety on her own, without the aid of drugs, and to face the events in her life that led her to be anxious. Since she and her psychiatrist were focusing on the wrong problem, it's no wonder that Susan never got better.

Susan wanted to stay on benzodiazepines, but some women who are dissatisfied with their effects may not want to challenge the doctor's advice, even if they don't like it, in order to preserve this connection. This, too, may lead them to stay on these drugs.

Benzodiazepines Blunt Anger

As anyone who works in a psychiatric ward knows, benzodiazepines are used to calm people down and lessen their anger—no matter what the problem is and no matter how angry the person is. For many women, the direct expression of anger was criticized by others as they grew up. They learn to repress feelings of anger and avoid expressing it because they think that other people won't like them. Using the self-in-relation theory, we can see that these women fear that expressing anger directly will disrupt the relationship. This fear kept Marilyn from disagreeing with her father's advice and confronting his domineering manner. It interfered with the ability of Susan and Heather to establish satisfactory relationships as adults. By blunting a woman's anger about some aspect of the relationship, benzodiazepines can help to preserve the appearance of harmony in a relationship even though the problems have not changed.

Benzodiazepines Remove Anxiety and the Urge to Change

These drugs allow relief from the anxiety that is caused by the internal conflict. When the feelings of anger and anxiety that would normally propel someone to try to change her situation are removed, so too is the motivation to address the problems. The relationship is preserved, but at the cost of continued unhappiness.

A woman's motivation to maintain the passive and dependent role that society, her spouse, parents, and boss have defined for her and restricted her to, and that she may have internalized as part of who she wants to be, may lead her to feel chronically inadequate when she feels things such as anger and aggression that she isn't "supposed" to feel. This feeling of inadequacy may lead her to take a pill to "fix" herself when she is anxious.

CONCLUSION

It is apparent that women take benzodiazepines more than men by a margin of two to one for many reasons, some of which are entwined with one another. Elderly women, who are prescribed these drugs at a rate higher than any other group, are especially vulnerable to these forces because they are more likely to have been socialized into a passive and dependent role in society than women of a more liberated age.

In my practice, I regularly see these factors affect the care that women receive. I see many more anxious women than men. Many have had previous treatment that aimed to help them stay in unsatisfying relationships. Some women have sought medicine from me to allow them to continue to blunt their feelings. Some women ask me nervously if it's okay with me that they make a change in their medication and even say that they are afraid I'll be mad at them for questioning my advice.

Self-in-relation theory has helped me to understand that many women find themselves in the Benzo Blues in an effort to maintain feelings of harmony in a relationship. It also points the way out of the Benzo Blues for many women. They become more willing to face the negative aspects of their use of these drugs and come off them when they learn that their medication promotes only a false harmony, and only at the cost of suppressing their true feelings. They come to see that any genuine closeness can grow only if they share those true feelings, and not just the pleasing ones.

In the next chapter we will look at an aspect of benzodiazepines we have ignored until now: their side effects.

· 7 ·

THE SIDE EFFECTS OF BENZOS

The term *side effect* is used to describe any effect other than the one for which the drug is used. Thus the main effect of a high-blood-pressure drug, for instance, is to lower blood pressure; other effects, such as lowered libido, are the drug's side effects. Usually side effects are merely annoying, such as stomach cramps or diarrhea from antibiotics. Sometimes, however, they can be more serious, like the ulcers that can occur with the use of antiinflammatory drugs like ibuprofen or naproxyn, or the decreased blood cell counts from drugs used in the treatment for cancer that can increase vulnerability to life-threatening infections.

Benzodiazepines do not cause toxic effects to other organs, such as the heart, lungs, gastrointestinal tract, liver, or kidneys. They can have many other effects, however, that must be taken into consideration in their use (see Table 2, p. 142). Although most people who prescribe or take these drugs know some of the side effects associated with short-term use, many people are unaware of the more subtle effects that can occur during long-term use.

People over sixty are relatively heavy users of benzodiazepines in relation to their representation in the general population.[1] They are especially sensitive to the drugs' side effects primarily because the liver breaks down these drugs much slower in the elderly, leading to higher blood levels for longer periods of time.[2] This leads the elderly to experience a higher rate of oversedation, memory impairment, cognitive confusion, and poor muscular coordination, which impairs driving ability and increases the rate of falls leading to hip fractures. Because elderly people may experience

TABLE 2

SIDE EFFECTS OF BENZODIAZEPINES

IMMEDIATE
  Sedation
  Poor muscle coordination
  Memory impairment
  Paradoxical reactions
  Miscellaneous

LONG-TERM
  Tolerance
  Emotional blunting
  Cognitive impairment
  Brain shrinkage

INDIRECT
  Effects in pregnant women
  Effects in other medical conditions
  Interactions with other drugs
  Falls and hip fractures
  Traffic accidents
  Overdose attempts and suicide completion
  Abuse

these problems from the aging process itself, the additive effects of benzodiazepines can lead to significantly impaired functioning.

I will first describe the side effects that occur in people when they start taking the drug, go on to discuss the impairments caused by long-term use, and then examine some of the indirect effects.

IMMEDIATE SIDE EFFECTS

Sedation

Although benzodiazepines are often called sedatives, their therapeutic effect of calming a person's anxiety is separate from their tendency to induce sedation, which is the feeling of fatigue that occurs when a person is tired. Sedation occurs commonly, although some cause more sedation than others because of differences in their chemical structures. For example, sedation occurs in sixteen percent of people who take Ativan, forty-one percent of those who take Xanax, and fifty percent of those who take Klonopin.[3]

The pronounced sedation caused by drugs such as Restoril, Dalmane, and Halcion has been effectively exploited by the pharmaceutical companies for use as sleeping aids. In this case, obviously, sedation is the therapeutic effect and is not a side effect at all. If the medication is being used primarily for the relief of anxiety during the day, however, then sedation is viewed primarily as a side effect. Sedation can impair a person's level of alertness, which can lead to decreased motivation and ability to perform tasks.

Poor Muscle Coordination

This class of drugs impairs performance on a variety of tests of physical coordination. These impairments can occur after both a single dose and repeated doses. Poor coordination is manifested at times by ataxia (unsteadiness of the feet) and dysarthria (slurred speech). Poor coordination is worse at higher doses. Muscle coordination in the elderly appears to be more easily impaired than that of younger patients.[4] As with sedation, the frequency of poor muscle coordination varies: 3.4 percent of people who take Ativan, 30 percent of those who take Klonopin, and forty percent of those who take Xanax.[5]

Memory Impairment

Benzodiazepines can cause anterograde amnesia, which means that people do not remember what happened for a few hours after they have taken a dose.[6] The degree of memory impairment depends on the dose and the route of administration, with higher doses and intravenous administration causing the greatest impairment. Older patients and those with a prior history of benzodiazepine use are more likely to experience memory impairment. Older subjects may experience an insidious gradual decrement in memory function even at constant doses.[7] Thirty percent of patients in one study reported memory deficits while on Xanax.[8] Experience with patients in my own practice suggests that this number under-estimates the actual frequency of memory impairment.

Paradoxical Reactions

Rarely, benzodiazepines can cause paradoxical excitement with in-creased anxiety, insomnia, nightmares, hallucinations at sleep onset, irritability, hyperactive or restless behavior, and seizures in epileptics.[9] Some patients who take alprazolam experience a form of behavioral dyscontrol, in which they are more likely to be im-pulsive and harm themselves.[10] There is no accepted estimate of the frequency of these effects, but my experience leads me to be-lieve they occur very infrequently. Paradoxical reactions generally resolve quickly and without adverse sequelae as soon as the drug is stopped.

Miscellaneous

Other effects that have been reported with benzodiazepine use in-clude double vision, vertigo, changes in libido, menstrual irregular-ities, incontinence, urinary retention, and dizziness.[11] These effects occur infrequently in patients who take these drugs.

SIDE EFFECTS ASSOCIATED WITH LONG-TERM USE

Tolerance

Physicians define tolerance as a condition in which a person gradu-ally experiences the effect of a medication in a less intense form the longer that they take the medication. Tolerance occurs as a result of the effects of a drug that cause changes in the body's cells and receptors that diminish the response of the cells to the drug in the future. Some of the tolerance to the effects of alcohol is because of this phenomenon. Tolerance can also be due to the way that the body absorbs, transports, metabolizes, and excretes a drug. For example, tolerance to alcohol, in which people need increasing amounts in order to get the same effect, is due partially to the higher rate of breakdown of alcohol by the liver in response to regular ingestion. Because the liver is chewing up the alcohol much faster, people need to drink more just to get the same amount to the brain.

Researchers disagree about whether or not people develop tolerance to the therapeutic effects benzodiazepines have on anxiety, in part because different investigators weigh different aspects of the clinical picture to reach their conclusions. Most researchers and clinicians have found that patients generally do not increase their dose as they stay on these drugs and some people even lower their dose a notch from the original dosage size if they stay on them for more than a few months. This leads many researchers and clinicians to feel that tolerance does not develop. Others feel that tolerance does develop because their research demonstrates that people continue to experience anxiety at the same level as before they started taking medication.

There is widespread agreement that tolerance develops quite quickly to the drugs' sedative effects.[12] Although daytime users of benzodiazepines may initially feel sleepy, this effect usually passes within a few days. The same thing happens with benzos used at night, however, as well.[13] This diminishing sedative effect at night renders the medication ineffective and allows insomnia to emerge.

People do not develop tolerance to the tendency of these drugs to impair memory.[14] Partial tolerance appears to develop to the impairment in physical coordination.

Emotional Blunting

Benzodiazepines diminish the intensity of anxiety and other feelings such as anger and sadness. Since some intense emotions can produce discomfort, this side effect may often be experienced as positive. However, patients who take benzodiazepines also experience less pleasure.

Heather Ashton, a British researcher who has written widely on the subject, reported that this "emotional anesthesia," or the inability to feel pleasure or pain, has similarities to the lack of ability to experience pleasure that is sometimes seen in depression. She notes that many long-term users who finally stop regret their lack of emotional response to events occurring during the period they were taking pills.[15]

I have noted in my own practice that not only do people notice a reemergence of many emotional feelings after tapering their usage, but they also often remark that they were unaware of the blunting while it was occurring.

Cognitive Impairment

Benzodiazepines cause cognitive impairment, which is when a person is less able to perform tasks requiring thinking.[16] Susan Golombok, a British researcher who has written several articles on the hazardous effects of benzodiazepines, found that their use for more than a year is associated with cognitive impairment in two areas.[17] The first is visual perceptual analysis, as measured by the ability of patients to perceive differences in complex designs. The second area of impairment is the ability to sustain attention on a repetitive task under time pressure. It appeared that taking a low dose for a short time had little effect on visual-spatial ability or sustained attention, while a high intake was almost certainly harmful. These two effects may have contributed to Jim's difficulty performing the detailed repetitive work with glass molds.

Most strikingly, Golombok also documents that patients are often unaware of their reduced ability. She reports that patients who withdrew from their medication often report improved concentration and increased sensory appreciation, and that only after withdrawal did they realize that they had been functioning below par.

Brain Shrinkage

In 1984, Malcolm Lader evaluated the sizes of different areas of the brain in twenty patients who had taken benzodiazepines for an average of more than ten years through evaluation of what was then a new radiological technique, the computerized tomography scan, or CT. Lader compared the CT scans of these users to CT scans of anxious people who had never taken these drugs. Lader reported that those who had taken the drugs demonstrated brain shrinkage, with enlargement of the fluid-filled spaces of the brain such as the ventricles, sulci, sylvian and interhemispheric fissures. The overall ventricle/brain ratio (VBR) of the benzodiazepine group was significantly larger than those of others.[18] This strongly suggests that there was a smaller brain mass in people who took these drugs for many years.

Since then, other studies have evaluated the possibility that long-term use causes brain shrinkage. One study of seventeen benzodiazepine-dependent patients found an elevated VBR when compared with an age- and sex-matched control group of people.[19] Another found an elevated VBR in a study of twenty-five patients with panic disorder who had used these drugs an average of three years.[20] On the other hand, one study was unable to confirm this finding in twenty-eight regular users.[21] Another study of nineteen patients found no difference between long-term users and controls.[22] No relationship was observed between VBR and previous treatment such as benzodiazepines in a study of patients with mood disorders or schizophrenia.[23]

The most careful study to date evaluated twenty-five subjects who had never taken benzodiazepines, nine subjects who had taken them in the past for less than one year, thirty patients who currently took them, and seventeen patients who had taken them in the past for at least one year but who had been withdrawn from medication for at least six months.[24] The brains of chronic users had decreased density in the right caudate nucleus, which is involved in the production of coordinated muscle movements, and the occipital areas bilaterally, which are responsible for processing of visual information. Those who took lorazepam (Ativan) had decreased density of the brain in the right caudate, left occipital, and both frontal lobes, which are involved in the process of abstract thinking. Those on diazepam (Valium) had no abnormalities. The investigators hypothesize that lorazepam users are receiving a consistently heavier load of benzodiazepine than diazepam users because lorazepam is often used at a higher equivalent dosage than diazepam.

These reports strongly suggest that the long-term use of benzodiazepines causes brain shrinkage in some patients, but the studies do not involve enough subjects to establish this beyond doubt. None of the authors speculate how benzodiazepines might cause this change, if indeed they do. There is no accepted understanding of how these changes might affect a person's ability to function, but given the impairments benzodiazepines cause to memory and cognition, these changes may have serious negative effects.

INDIRECT EFFECTS

Effects of Benzodiazepines in Pregnant Women and People with Other Medical Conditions

Benzodiazepines cross the placenta and, if taken regularly by a mother in late pregnancy, can cause neonatal complications. For example, babies may experience withdrawal symptoms after birth, showing irritability and feeding difficulties. For two weeks after birth, infants born to mothers who use these drugs regularly may experience the "floppy infant syndrome," which consists of poor muscle tone, failure to suck, and central nervous system depression.[25] Regular use even in therapeutic doses may impair intrauterine growth.[26] There is a slightly higher rate of babies born with a cleft palate to women who take benzodiazepines.[27] A higher incidence of birth defects occurs in women who simultaneously use a high dose of benzodiazepines and also abuse drugs and alcohol, but this may not be due to the benzodiazepines.[28]

People with impairment of their liver function metabolize benzodiazepines more slowly, leading to higher blood levels of the drugs than usual from therapeutic doses. This can lead them to experience some of the other side effects, such as sedation and poor coordination, at lower doses than usual.

People with impaired breathing due to respiratory illness can experience an exacerbation of their breathing problems on benzodiazepines.

Interactions with Other Drugs

By and large, the effects of benzodiazepines with most other drugs is negligible. However, their use can lead to increased sedative effects if combined with drugs that cause some central nervous system depression, including anticonvulsants such as Luminol, Depakote, Dilantin, and Tegretol; antihistamines such as Benadryl; neuroleptics such as Thorazine and Mellaril; and antidepressants such as Elavil and Pamelor.

Benzodiazepines can cause pronounced psychomotor impairment and oversedation in combination with alcohol. Although even large doses rarely cause death if no other drugs are taken, fatalities have occurred with the combined use of alcohol and an overdose of these drugs.

Falls and Hip Fractures

Falls are a leading cause of accidental death in people more than sixty-five years of age in the United States.[29] They contribute to forty percent of nursing home admissions. Five percent of falls result in hip fractures and other injuries that require hospitalization or immobilization for an extended period.[30] It is apparent that falls and hip fractures are a major health problem for the elderly and a major cost issue for society.

The elderly have both a higher risk of falling and a higher rate of hip fractures when taking benzodiazepines.[31] In one study involving more than 6,000 patients, those taking flurazepam, diazepam, or chlordiazepoxide had a risk of hip fracture 1.8 times greater than those not taking this class of drugs.[32] Another study evaluated 336 people seventy-five or older living in the community and found that the use of sedatives such as benzos, antidepressants, and antipsychotics increased the rate of falls.[33] A third study found that there were 507 falls in 761 subjects monitored for one year. Use of hypnotics or any other psychiatric medication such as antidepressants was associated with an increased rate of falls.[34] A fourth compared 100 patients in a hospital who had fallen and 100 controls who had not, all seventy years of age or older, and found that a higher rate of falls was associated with benzodiazepine use.[35]

Traffic Accidents

Benzos impair specific driving skills such as the ability to regulate speed, lane position, and passing and parking, although these effects are not consistent from person to person and may depend on when a dose is taken. The APA Task Force reports that this class of drugs "probably" impairs driving skills mostly in older persons and in those who have not previously taken such drugs, although repeated regular therapeutic doses do not impair automobile driving skills in most people.[36]

Other research articles have reached more troubling conclusions. The risk of a traffic accident rises after patients are given a prescription for benzodiazepines, and those who filled three prescriptions in a six-month period had an even higher risk.[37] Another study of over 300,000 people found that the risk of a traffic accident was significantly greater for people who had received a prescription than for controls. The risk was highest during the first week after the prescription was filled but remained higher even four weeks later.[38] A third study of 16,000 drivers over the age of sixty-five found that the risk of an accident was significantly higher in those taking benzos.[39]

Overdose Attempts and Suicide Completions

Benzodiazepines are used in excessive amounts in suicide attempts. In one study there were 5.9 deaths per million prescriptions written, with an estimated rate of forty-seven deaths per million patients prescribed benzos.[40] It is important to note that the frequency of prescriptions and overdoses from these drugs decreased during a public relations campaign in Sweden from 1978 to 1981 to decrease the frequency of their being prescribed. After the campaign stopped, the rate of prescription and rate of overdose again rose.[41] A lower rate of overdosage was also noted in New York State when the rate of benzodiazepine prescriptions dropped because of state regulations.[42]

Abuse

A very small portion of people use benzodiazepines for nonmedical reasons.[43] Sometimes they obtain a prescription by misrepresenting their symptoms to a physician, but they often purchase benzodiazepines illegally on the street. In general, people who seek inappropriate access to this class of drugs for recreational usage also abuse other drugs. Opiate users sometimes use them to strengthen their euphoria. People who abuse cocaine and amphetamines sometimes use them to come down from their high more gradually. Thirty to forty percent of alcohol abusers take benzodiazepines.[44] Valium, Xanax, and Ativan are most likely to be used.[45] One review stated that some people have abused Restoril by injection, with complications that include withdrawal convulsions, deep vein thrombosis, gangrene, and death.[46]

The prevailing attitude of the medical profession and patients alike is that benzodiazepines cause minimal side effects. It is true that most people do not find the short-term side effects significantly troubling. However, memory difficulties, cognitive impairment, emotional blunting, brain shrinkage, hip fractures, and traffic accidents associated with long-term use cause considerable distress and injury to patients, especially to the elderly, and are a great cost to society. These complications have been virtually ignored by many in the medical community and downplayed by others. Given that long-term usage has not been proven to help anxiety, the lack of recognizing the importance of these effects is all the more troubling. The possibility that long-term use leads to brain shrinkage is especially troubling and has not received the attention it deserves by the medical profession.

Some of the reasons that people avoid recognizing the complications of long-term use were discussed in chapter 4: Patients are desperate for relief; doctors want to help; drug companies want to make money; and third-party payers want to blanket feelings with drugs as the cheapest solution. The stigma against mental illness plays the most important role, however. Everyone wants to see patients "appear" normal rather than acknowledge how they truly are: anxious, overwhelmed, and in pain about events and situations in their life. Everyone wants to pretend that things aren't too bad and that the symptoms are just a bothersome aberration.

Benzodiazepines allow a person to maintain a false front that masquerades as reality. Recognizing unpleasant and even dangerous side effects detracts from building and maintaining this false front, however, which is one reason people are loath to do it. Maintaining this front has led to tremendous personal distress at an enormous cost to society.

Given all these problems, is the use of benzodiazepines ever wise? In the next chapter we will see that they can be used sensibly in the treatment of many medical and psychiatric disorders.

· 8 ·

WHEN *CAN* BENZOS BE USEFUL?

The thesis of this book is that benzodiazepines should not be used for treatment of chronic anxiety. Due to their sedative effects and the relatively low incidence of short-term side effects, however, they have been widely applied in a variety of medical and psychiatric disorders. In this chapter we will look at their use for anxiety and in these other conditions.

ANXIETY DISORDERS

As the previous three chapters have demonstrated, there are few hard facts that provide clear guidance about how to use benzodiazepines. Given this lack of clear guidelines, the most sensible approach is to identify each aspect of a person's symptoms of anxiety and the circumstances in life that contribute to the anxiety, and develop a comprehensive treatment plan that addresses each one. The decision of whether or not to use these drugs can be sensibly made only after weighing their risks and benefits as they apply to the person's unique circumstances and the overall treatment plan. A complete treatment plan that addresses a patient's symptoms, distress, and the current and past issues that led to the present anxiety can only be formulated after this evaluation. The decision whether or not to use benzodiazepines must be part of the overall plan to accomplish the goals of treatment. They are not the treatment plan itself.

The Elements of a Complete Evaluation of Anxiety

A complete evaluation has many components. There is no easy shortcut to deciding how to help someone with anxiety and whether benzodiazepines might be useful. An hour-long interview is generally necessary to learn the relevant information, reach a shared understanding with the patient about the problems, and outline an initial treatment plan.

PATIENT CHARACTERISTICS. It is essential that the physician know some basic facts about a person's life in order to place any difficulties with anxiety in some context. The influence of a person's gender was discussed in chapter 6, but there are many others as well.

Age. Anxiety about open spaces in a thirty-year-old is quite different from anxiety about leaving the house in a seventy-year-old. Active, young, and midlife adults are generally self-sufficient, and the impairment caused by agoraphobia can have a much more pronounced effect on them than on the elderly. This impairment needs to be addressed directly in order to enable the patient to regain confidence in his ability to function. The elderly often have thoughts about their own death that significantly influence their anxiety about an unresolved part of their life and their willingness to pursue different treatment options. Some are intent on pushing themselves to overcome any limitation placed on them by medical problems or physical weakness by such means as dieting or exercise; others are more willing to accept limitations and gain a sense of calm and peacefulness as they continue to confront the issues of age.

Culture. Patients from different cultural backgrounds can have different symptoms of anxiety and different expectations about the usefulness of medications. For example, some people of Asian heritage are ashamed to express any psychological distress and may cover their distress and anxiety about issues in their life by first discussing medical complaints. Suggestions that they might need medication can be experienced as an insult because it implies that there is something wrong with them. At the same time, they may follow the doctor's recommendations to the letter even if they disagree, because they don't want to insult someone in authority. It is important to spend time with all patients to understand exactly how they wish to be treated before making any recommendations that they will feel obliged to follow.

Family History. Do other members of the patient's family experience intense anxiety? If so, who, what kind, for how long, what treatments did they try, and what worked for them? Although we may not yet be able to identify any specific biological vulnerability to anxiety, treatments useful for one member of a family can often be helpful for another.

Marital Status. To a sufferer, it may seem that their anxiety does not affect other people, and it may even make them feel more cut off from others. However, this is rarely true. For those who are married, their partner is also being affected by their anxiety. It is essential for the doctor to understand the role of the partner in a person's anxiety. A supportive or conflicted relationship can affect the onset of anxiety and the usefulness of any treatment. For example, couples therapy may be necessary if one of the contributing factors to a person's anxiety includes problems between the partners, such as communication difficulties or unresolved issues from the past. Even if there are no major problems between a person with anxiety and his partner, it can be enormously helpful to meet with a partner a couple of times to gain support for the use of psychotherapy with its inevitable ups and downs, and to help them to see that the relief afforded by benzodiazepines is illusory.

Employment. The nature of how a person obtains support financially must also be assessed. If the patient doesn't work at all, is this due to anxiety? The nature of a person's job and the relationship with her boss must be understood to assess the impact of anxiety in this area of a person's life. Do symptoms interfere with work, as Susan experienced? If work causes the anxiety, is it the work itself, as might be the case for a nurse, fireman, or teacher, or is the trouble caused by circumstances of the job, such as an overly demanding boss? It may be that the anxiety is due to stresses at the job that need to be addressed by changing the work environment rather than by providing psychiatric treatment of medications or psychotherapy.

Other Medical Problems. Hyperthyroidism can cause symptoms of anxiety and needs to be ruled out by carefully questioning the patient about the other symptoms of a thyroid disorder and by blood tests if necessary. I have seen many patients who complained of anxiety with palpitations and shortness of breath who actually had cardiac and respiratory problems. Other medical conditions that produce symptoms that can be confused with anxiety include Cushing's disease and hypoglycemia. A pheochromocytoma, a tumor of the adrenal gland that produces excessive epinephrine, can cause symptoms that mimic panic attacks.

SYMPTOM CHARACTERISTICS. It is essential, obviously, to understand the characteristics of a person's symptoms of anxiety in order to arrive at a correct diagnosis. Is the anxiety a continuous phenomenon, or does it come in discrete panic attacks? Is the person more troubled in certain places? Is he awakened at night by nightmares? Is the distress primarily caused by rituals that interfere with functioning? Once the general outlines of a specific anxiety disorder come into view, the physician must confirm the initial hypothesis by inquiring about all the symptoms of that specific disorder. For example, occasional nightmares about a difficult experience is not sufficient reason to give someone a diagnosis of PTSD; the patient must be attempting to avoid stimuli associated with the trauma and experiencing symptoms of increased arousal.

The intensity of the symptoms must also be evaluated. Some people are moderately troubled by panic attacks, while others are truly overwhelmed. People can have varying degrees of compulsions with OCD. The intensity of the symptoms can influence the choice of treatment. Overwhelming distress needs to be addressed immediately, a role in which benzodiazepines can be very useful, whereas milder anxiety may respond to psychotherapy alone. The duration of symptoms is important, too. For instance, the description of their war experiences given to me in 1978 by two veterans sounded very similar except for one factor: one had served in Vietnam four years earlier, and the other had served in World War II more than thirty years earlier. The older veteran had a far lengthier experience of nightmares, flashbacks, anxiety, and rage and, as a result, had a much more rigid coping style. This style led him to be far less amenable to psychotherapy.

CURRENT STRESSES. It is essential to explore all areas of a person's current life that may be contributing to her anxiety in order to build on her strengths and positive aspects. These include the areas we have just discussed as well as her sexual life, spiritual beliefs, early experiences in life that have shaped the choices that were made, satisfaction with life, and goals for the future. It is important to evaluate whether shifts in the developmental stages of life, such as moving away from one's parents, the search for intimacy with others, the birth of children, or changes due to aging are contributing to anxiety.

The current stresses that lead to anxiety are not always so clear. For example, the departure of children from the home can be a difficult transition for many parents, but the distress may start long before the last child actually leaves.

PAST STRESSES/TRAUMA. I cannot emphasize strongly enough that an exploration of a person's childhood experience is essential in order to put any current symptoms into the proper perspective. Most of the people I've described were prescribed benzodiazepines for what appeared to be straightforward anxiety about current problems. Unfortunately, they became ensnared in the Benzo Blues because they had been struggling with anxiety due to experiences from earlier in their life that no one had ever helped them address.

Initially, patients often deny obvious traumas such as sexual or physical abuse because they are painful and embarrassing. The physician must use tact and take the time to bring up potentially painful subjects in a manner that allows patients to acknowledge their traumas, what they meant to them, and what they can do to get some help at this late date. More subtle traumas, such as emotional abuse, the effects of divorce, or the effects of being raised by parents who abused alcohol, may require an extended period of time to fully understand because over time more and more memories start to emerge, raising long-buried feelings.

PREVIOUS TREATMENT AND COPING METHODS. How has a person coped thus far with psychological distress? Has she restricted herself, like Marilyn and Debbie? Has she generally resorted to medications like Susan? Does he know, use, or practice any relaxation techniques? Has he ever been in psychotherapy? If so, what did he learn? The answers to these questions are essential to guide any treatment recommendations. It is pointless to recommend treatments that have previously failed and highly useful to know what may have worked in the past.

This is where the inadequacy of benzodiazepines often first becomes clear. Not only do people taking them rarely use other treatment methods, but they also continue to struggle with anxiety. Explaining that there are other treatments for anxiety besides medication can be helpful to people who don't want to rely on drugs but who don't know what else to do.

SUBSTANCE ABUSE. Many people who suffer with anxiety use alcohol, marijuana, and other drugs. Someone with anxiety who is, for example, using alcohol more often than occasionally should raise the concern that the drug is being used to calm anxiety. Other treatment methods invariably fail when a person uses controlled substances for relief because he is always looking for the next time to use a drug that will provide that relief. It is essential to clarify a person's alcohol and drug use to insure that it is adequately addressed in the treatment plan. Nor need the subject be confined to controlled substances. Caffeine and nicotine use can make symptoms of anxiety worse. People who drink six cups of coffee a day can often experience significant relief from anxiety just by switching to a decaffeinated brand.

PERSONAL VIEW OF THE PATIENT. No matter what treatment seems appropriate to the professional, it is essential to acknowledge and discuss a patient's own assessment of the stresses that are causing anxiety, preferences for treatment, and motivation to engage in different treatments.

We know that many people with anxiety are not aware of what is leading to their anxiety, but how can treatment take place without this knowledge? I try to reach in the first session at least some tentative ideas about the sources of a person's anxiety. Although we may revise these ideas as we spend more time examining a person's life, it gives us a sensible place to start. For example, Susan initially stated that her anxiety came out of nowhere, but even in the first session with me she was able to acknowledge that it started as she was becoming more deeply involved with Mark, her first serious boyfriend. It is unfortunate that many people are started on medications without coming even to some tentative agreement about what the causes are.

Most people are much more willing to follow a course of treatment if it coincides with their own preferences, so it's essential to find out what those preferences are. Knowing what those preferences are can also highlight forms of treatment that the patient may be reluctant to pursue.

I often recommend treatment about which people are initially hesitant because it seems lengthier and more difficult than just taking a pill. I always assess the patient's motivation to try treatment methods that may be difficult but effective before recommending any treatment because some people may need a detailed explanation of forms of treatment that they know little about, such as relaxation techniques and psychotherapy. They may also need additional encouragement to try something that is new to them.

The Assessment of Anxiety

After I have completed an evaluation of someone with anxiety, I assess whether the difficulties are most accurately seen as a crisis, as an acute syndrome, or as a chronic problem. Not surprisingly, the use of benzodiazepines differs depending on which one of the three best explains the anxiety.

ANXIETY IN A CRISIS. Sudden catastrophic events such as a death, physical illness, being fired, or being involved in a natural disaster such as an earthquake can overwhelm many people who otherwise function quite well. Psychotherapy alone is often sufficient to take care of the problem, but benzodiazepines can sometimes help people to function more effectively during these events by decreasing the intensity of their emotions. Their use for both sedation at night and anxiety relief during the day can be reasonable. The risk of developing an ongoing dependence on benzodiazepines is minimal[1] even if the event is truly catastrophic.[2]

It is important to evaluate whether or not the event is one that is truly out of the ordinary for the individual, or whether they have been functioning with chronic anxiety all along. Marilyn had exactly this kind of experience. Her husband's death led her to experience overt anxiety leading to the use of benzodiazepines. In fact, however, she had been functioning with significant anxiety even before her husband's death. In general, people who have learned how to manage their anxiety effectively do not use these drugs for more than a few doses, no matter how overwhelming the interpersonal event.

ACUTE ANXIETY. Whereas a crisis can overwhelm anyone temporarily, acute anxiety occurs when a person's anxiety is more intense or lasts longer than is warranted by the stresses in their life. This can be the case with an adjustment disorder or acute stress disorder, specific phobia, or the start of panic disorder, agoraphobia, generalized anxiety disorder, obsessive-compulsive disorder, and anxiety disorder, not otherwise specified (people with social phobia generally experience lifelong anxiety and rarely notice any acute onset).

Sometimes people feel intensely anxious when flying on an airplane or undergoing an uncomfortable medical procedure such as an MRI brain scan. It often makes sense to prescribe a benzodiazepine to help them through the situation with as little discomfort as possible. As long as they do not experience anxiety in other parts of their life, there is little risk of ongoing dependence.

There is no specific time period that differentiates acute from chronic anxiety. In general, acute anxiety has lasted or will be expected to last a matter of weeks to months. More important than the time period involved is whether the person continues attempts to overcome the symptoms and hold on to her view of herself as a person who can master the anxiety and move on in life or whether she begins to accommodate to the anxiety. Accommodation implies that the person expects to be anxious indefinitely. When the shift to accommodation has occurred—and this can happen within some weeks—the anxiety is most effectively treated with a long-term approach.

Many people with acute anxiety are able to manage the symptoms through the use of intensive psychotherapy, relaxation training, and support from family and friends. However, some people are genuinely overwhelmed and may need the cushion of a couple of weeks of benzodiazepines while they are contacting and meeting their therapists, learning about relaxation techniques, and perhaps using other medications.

Some patients with posttraumatic stress disorder can benefit from a brief course of benzodiazepines if the memories become especially acute because of work they are doing in therapy. Some people with GAD, OCD, and ADNOS can also experience intense exacerbations of their symptoms as a result of other stresses in their life for which a short course of benzodiazepines (less than two weeks) can be helpful. One must be careful not to prescribe them for too long and start up a dependency that is difficult to stop.

CHRONIC ANXIETY. I am opposed to the long-term use of benzodiazepines even in people with chronic anxiety—anxiety that has continued long after an acute crisis and become an ongoing part of a person's life. So the question remains, is their extended use ever justified?

I never prescribe benzodiazepines for someone with chronic anxiety who is not currently taking them with the intention of maintaining the prescription indefinitely. As Lader emphasized in 1993, no new long term users should be created.[3] Other medications and other treatment methods detailed in Section II help people with long-term anxiety far more in the long run.

The problem really arises when someone has already been getting benzodiazepines for years and still wants them. Such patients often have no idea of how these drugs are sabotaging their lives and generally plead with me to continue their prescription. I try to help them to see that the drugs have not helped them manage their anxiety and work with them to gradually discontinue them. This can be a long, difficult, and often contentious process. Some people refuse this work. If a patient is adamant about staying on benzodiazepines, I generally suggest that they seek out a physician who is willing to continue to prescribe them. It is unfortunate that all too many physicians go along with such a request.

Over the last ten years, however, there have been some people whom I have continued on benzodiazepines, sometimes against my better judgment, because I can think of no useful alternative. Although I have seen hundreds and hundreds of people use them on a long term basis, this group of "exceptions" numbers fewer than ten. I look at the following factors to evaluate whether benzodiazepines may be indicated for somebody who is experiencing anxiety.

Age. Many elderly patients are able to stop their benzodiazepines,[4] and it is important not to write them off as too old to change. I have seen many senior citizens get off them, especially those who use them primarily for sleep. Others have experienced anxiety for fifty, sixty, and even seventy years and are unwilling to pursue other forms of treatment. Some feel that they are incapable of making use of relaxation techniques or psychotherapy. Although I may disagree with their assessment of their ability to change, I respect their success in meeting life's challenges as well as they have. It therefore seems reasonable to consider long-term use in patients who have had anxiety for many decades, who are unwilling or incapable of engaging in other treatment, and in whom withdrawal of the medication would cause such distress that hospitalization might be required.

Severity of Symptoms. Some patients with posttraumatic stress disorder and obsessive-compulsive disorder can experience such intensity of symptoms that even years of therapy, practice in relaxation techniques, and the use of other medications are only minimally effective. If the severity of symptoms are such that they would cause hospitalization, and benzodiazepines can prevent that, then consideration should be given to continuing to write a prescription.

Current Stresses. Some people with an anxiety disorder are under significant stress in their real life for a prolonged time. For example, people with posttraumatic stress disorder resulting from sexual abuse or rape may experience prolonged stress if they are called to testify against the perpetrator. There are often numerous court delays with no resolution in sight. Although not ideal by any means, prolonged use of a benzodiazepine until the situation is resolved may be the best available alternative. However, once the court case is finished or the stress has passed, the drug should be tapered and stopped.

Other Treatments. I am uncomfortable prescribing benzodiazepines for long periods of time to people who have not previously engaged in other forms of treatment, including taking other medications, rigorously practicing relaxation techniques, and engaging in individual or group psychotherapy. Many people who initially feel they are unable to get off these drugs find that they are able to do so with relative ease once they have begun to effectively use other forms of treatment.

Rarely, people have had such severe difficulties in their life with anxiety that they have tried any number of treatments over the years in a genuine and serious fashion with only minimal benefit. For people who have engaged in all other forms of treatment without relief, benzodiazepines as the last resort may be a reasonable option.

A Person's Wishes. Although most longtime users initially express hesitation about stopping, many would like to if only they knew how. Some people have a strong wish to stay on benzodiaze-pines, and have no desire whatsoever to get off them. Although a desire to stay on them is not sufficient to me to continue the prescription, it is one factor that certainly needs to be considered.

Having discussed the elements of a good patient evaluation of anxiety and when to use benzodiazepines, there are some other conditions for which they may be an appropriate treatment.

INSOMNIA

Besides anxiety, insomnia is the most common reason that people take benzodiazepines. There is almost unanimous agreement among researchers, clinicians, and patients alike that these drugs effectively induce sleep for the first several nights.

Interestingly, most research has shown that their beneficial ef-fects for sleep wane over some weeks.[5] Many patients who have taken them for many months or even years feel that they are un-able to sleep without the pills, however. The difference between what is reported in the scientific literature and the subjective expe-rience of people who take benzodiazepines was examined in a 1988 study of forty people with chronic insomnia who had been on ben-zodiazepines for six months or more and felt unable to stop the drug even though they wanted to.[6] These users were compared with thirty-six people with chronic insomnia who did not take sleeping aids. After initial evaluations comparing the two groups, patients who had been prescribed benzodiazepines stopped taking them and a further comparison was made. The evaluation of the sleep of these groups of patients was done with polysomnographic recordings throughout the entire night, as well as subjective evalu-ation of sleep by all the patients.

Sleep duration was the same in both groups. However, REM sleep was significantly reduced in people who took benzodiazepines. REM sleep is the period of sleep in which people dream, and it plays an important restorative role in overall day-to-day functioning. When people stopped taking their medication, sleep duration increased in twenty-one patients and decreased in nineteen patients, and there was a dramatic increase of REM sleep in all forty of the patients. Interestingly, patients overestimated the amount of time they slept when they took the benzodiazepines and underestimated the time that they slept after the drugs were withdrawn.

Withdrawal insomnia appeared to be more a matter of perception rather than part of the sleep process itself. The unpleasant experience in coming off a benzodiazepine is often based on a patient's awareness of sleep disturbances when he stops it. Patients who use benzodiazepines every night and claim continued efficacy may in fact be experiencing some anterograde amnesia, so that they do not remember how long they stayed awake before they actually did fall asleep.

Insomnia rarely exists in a vacuum. Sufferers generally have other psychiatric disorders that are leading them to feel distress, such as schizophrenia, bipolar disorder, depression, or anxiety. Other causes of nighttime insomnia include alcohol or caffeine use, daily naps, medical disorders such as hyperthyroidism, sleep apnea, cardiac and respiratory problems. It is important, therefore, to undertake a full investigation of what could be contributing to insomnia before suggesting any specific treatment. It is unfortunately the case that many people are prescribed sleeping pills when they complain of insomnia, but the underlying disorder, which is causing the insomnia, goes untreated.

Because of the problems associated with tolerance and withdrawal, and because of the long-term ineffectiveness of benzodiazepines, I limit their use to four weeks for people who experience chronic insomnia. This is consistent with recommendations by most medical authorities.[7] Behavioral treatments have been shown to result in permanent improvement in people's ability to fall and stay asleep and feel more satisfied with their sleep.[8]

Other medications can be useful in the treatment of chronic insomnia without the long-term negative effects of benzodiazepines and without a gradual loss of effectiveness. Desyrel, which is sometimes used as an antidepressant, generally causes moderate sedation at even small dosages, and this side effect can be effectively exploited for people who experience chronic insomnia. There are no significant long-term negative effects to Desyrel that we are currently aware of, and the drug does not appear to lose its effectiveness. The recently released Ambien appears to be effective for extended periods of time without negative effects. However, it has not been in use very long, and there is insufficient documentation in the scientific literature to establish its efficacy for long-term use.

OTHER PSYCHIATRIC AND MEDICAL CONDITIONS

Benzodiazepines can improve sleep and decrease agitation during the day in a person with *depression*. This can be an enormous relief, and often some transient improvement occurs in the depression itself. In general, insomnia and agitation resolve in some weeks with proper treatment of the depression. The relief can be a trap, however, for if the benzodiazepines are continued week after week, they can contribute to a person's depression, sense of hopelessness, and lack of motivation to change as they slide into the Benzo Blues.

They can be helpful for people with *bipolar disorder* (manic-depressive illness) in three ways. They can calm a person who is acutely agitated in the midst of a manic episode. They can also prevent future manic episodes when taken regularly. Finally, a manic episode often starts with sleeplessness, and a prescription of a benzodiazepine to ensure adequate sleep often minimizes the intensity of the episode and occasionally averts it entirely.

Although benzodiazepines have no specific antipsychotic effect, they are sometimes used in the treatment of *schizophrenia* to help patients feel some relief from the never-ending onslaught of their hallucinations and delusions. Antipsychotic drugs used to combat the symptoms of schizophrenia often cause akathisia, a restlessness that is relieved primarily by walking. Benzodiazepines significantly lessen the intensity of akathisia.

Librium and Serax are commonly prescribed by physicians in the treatment of *alcohol withdrawal* to prevent delirium tremens (DTs), seizures, and even death. The period of time that a benzodiazepine is needed to prevent serious complications from alcohol withdrawal varies, depending on the amount and duration of alcohol use, but a few days to a week is usually sufficient. People who take benzodiazepines longer than two weeks following cessation of alcohol are using it primarily for its effects on their anxiety, not for its prevention of DTs or seizures. Some long-term users began their use when they were getting off alcohol, and both they and their physician saw it as a better alternative. The substitution of benzodiazepines for alcohol changes the external form of the addiction and gives it the veneer of respectability because of the MD's authority. Nevertheless, maintaining such an addiction is a poor plan—abstinence should be the goal.

Benzodiazepines are also used for *muscle spasms, epilepsy,* and for *preanesthesia* relaxation prior to a surgical procedure.

In summary, there are many good reasons to prescribe benzodiazepines. Used carefully and sensibly, they can provide enormous relief of anxiety and other symptoms of distress in a wide variety of situations. The benefits that they provide in these conditions contribute to their reputation as safe and effective drugs and to their inappropriate use in chronic anxiety. In contrast to patients who use benzodiazepines in these other conditions, however, those with chronic anxiety often become dependent on them and ensnared into the Benzo Blues. In the next section we will see how such people are able to stop their usage, master their anxiety, and take charge of their life.

Part ◆ Two

HOW TO STOP BENZOS AND START LEADING YOUR LIFE AGAIN

I gain strength, courage, and confidence by every experience in which I must stop and look fear in the face. . . . I say to myself, I've lived through this and can take the next thing that comes along. . . . We must do the things we cannot do.

—Eleanor Roosevelt

· 9 ·

EFFECTIVE TREATMENTS FOR ANXIETY

If the thought of getting off your pills scares you, it is probably due in part to your concern that you don't know how you are going to tolerate the symptoms of anxiety—panic attacks, restlessness, sleepless nights, etc. However, there are many other treatments for anxiety besides benzodiazepines, and three have been found to be especially effective: relaxation techniques, medications, and psychotherapy. Each has helped millions of people.

You may also be nervous because you've previously been involved in treatment for anxiety that was ineffective. This can occur when significant elements that contributed to your anxiety, such as early-life issues, are ignored and continue to cause you anxiety. Perhaps your treatment was not meticulously planned, with methods chosen primarily because they were preferred by your doctor, rather than because they were appropriate for you and the unique circumstances that led to your anxiety. Perhaps your treatment was incomplete, which can occur if your doctor used inadequate dosages of medication. Or perhaps you got discouraged and didn't practice relaxation techniques vigorously or gave up on psychotherapy before you got any benefit out of it.

A sound treatment plan for getting off benzodiazepines requires that you consult a psychiatrist who knows how to perform a full evaluation. Most other physicians do not have the training or the time to make a comprehensive assessment of psychiatric disorders and are often unfamiliar with effective treatment methods such as psychotherapy. The plan you and a psychiatrist develop should take your unique experience of anxiety into account and employ methods to address each problem area. It will require a good collaboration between the two of you so that you both agree on the problems and the methods chosen to help you. Any good treatment plan requires your active participation to be successful: as you'll see, you can't just "follow doctor's orders." A good plan also needs ongoing input from your psychiatrist in helping you overcome the inevitable roadblocks and setbacks.

Some third-party payers refuse to pay psychiatrists to perform psychotherapy, maintaining that other mental health professionals can do so at a lower cost. It is reasonable to split the treatment between a psychiatrist who performs the initial evaluation and then monitors the medication throughout the course of treatment and a psychotherapist such as a social worker or psychologist who performs the psychotherapy, as long as the psychiatrist, psychotherapist, and patient agree with the overall plan and communicate effectively when problems arise. The most common problem occurs when the patient feels increased anxiety because of issues that arise in therapy and calls the psychiatrist to prescribe medications for relief. Good communication between the therapist and psychiatrist at this point can help the patient address the issue in its proper place—i.e., psychotherapy sessions—rather than engage in merely blunting the anxiety with medication.

It is important to understand that the following description and summary of effective treatment methods for reducing the symptoms of anxiety are no more effective a treatment plan for you and your anxiety than is a prescription for benzodiazepines. Rather, they are described here to provide you with some knowledge about other treatment methods that have been helpful to other people and that you may want to include in your plan.

RELAXATION TECHNIQUES

When you and your psychiatrist taper your benzodiazepine usage, you will experience intensified symptoms of anxiety as part of withdrawal. You will need to have an alternative to taking benzodiazepines to help you tolerate this intensification when it occurs. Whether primarily physical or psychological in nature, relaxation techniques—deliberately chosen exercises to minimize the physical effects of anxiety—can help you to achieve and maintain a feeling of calm when your dosage is reduced and in anxiety-provoking situations. Although the ability to stay calm won't change the circumstances that lead you to be anxious, it will allow you to face situations with a new sense of confidence that you will not be betrayed by your own body.

The development of relaxation techniques derives from the work of Herbert Benson, a cardiologist at Harvard. He described his discoveries in his classic book, *The Relaxation Response* (1975).[1] Benson knew that involuntary bodily processes, such as the pulse, blood pressure, the frequency of intestinal contractions, and the amount of blood flowing to a particular region of the body could be altered in animals in response to environmental cues.[2] In an effort to help people with hypertension, Benson took this phenomenon a step further. He devised a system that would "feed back" information about blood pressure to laboratory monkeys, training them to raise or lower their blood pressure through a system of rewards and punishments. He was then able to accomplish this same result in humans. His human subjects informed him that they could lower their blood pressure by thinking relaxing thoughts.

About this time, devotees of transcendental meditation (TM) approached Benson and requested that he study them, because they could lower their blood pressure through meditation. TM is derived from the classic form of meditation used by Buddhists and Hindus, who perform it in order to improve spiritual development. The meditation is performed with the person sitting on the ground with legs crossed, arms in a relaxed position, eyes open and fixed on a specific object. The aim is to attain a relaxed body, with slowed breathing, and an absence of thought about day-to-day matters. Devotees generally practice daily for many years to attain proficiency at meditation and gain spiritual enlightenment.

As imported into the West by the Maharishi Mahesh Yogi in the sixties, TM combined the Eastern method of meditation for spiritual enlightenment with the West's penchant for easy success. Rather than spending years learning the classic form of Eastern meditation, practitioners of TM could achieve serenity with just two daily twenty-minute periods of meditation in which they concentrated on a special word, or mantra, given to them by their teacher. Although the popularity of TM waxed and waned rather quickly, its practitioners noted a surprising alteration in their physiology—measurably lowered blood pressure.

At that time, the idea that meditation could affect blood pressure was thought to be impossible by Western medical authorities. They contended that alteration in a person's state of mind could not exert any effects on the autonomic nervous system. Benson agreed to study practitioners of TM and found that their claim was true—they *could* lower their blood pressure through meditation. He demonstrated that other forms of meditation could lower blood pressure as well. He also discovered that besides lower blood pressure, meditation could cause other physiological changes, including a state of increased calm, a lower heart rate, lower oxygen consumption, decreased muscle tension, and increased alpha waves in the brain. He termed the effect the Relaxation Response. Benson realized that many people, not just those with hypertension, could derive benefit from his discovery.

In *The Relaxation Response,* Benson recommended regular practice of relaxation techniques not for spiritual advancement or even to lower hypertension, but as a method to help people maintain an inner state of calm in their lives. In his book he described a relaxation technique that eliminates the spiritual aspects of the meditation experience but maintains the core elements that induce the physical response, including the maintenance of a comfortable position, regular breathing, and meditation on a single word or mantra, such as *one.*

Many other relaxation techniques have been developed since the publication of Benson's book. The common advice to "take a deep breath" when stressed is in fact a description of a brief relaxation technique that allows the person to relax the body physically. People with chronic anxiety, however, need to practice relaxation techniques more deliberately in order to maintain the same level of relaxation that others are able to reach by simply "taking a deep breath."

The goal of all relaxation techniques is to enable a person to achieve a sense of relaxation in a calm situation and then gradually generalize that ability to situations that would normally provoke anxiety. Following are brief descriptions of six different relaxation methods that people have found helpful.

Many people find their initial attempts to practice the techniques frustrating because they experience even greater anxiety than usual when they attempt to just sit quietly. Using relaxation tapes to provide an external soothing force initially can be helpful. It is imperative to keep practicing the other techniques, however, since otherwise the internal skill to relax will not develop. Most people I've worked with find the breathing and progressive muscular relaxation techniques to be the most useful. Not only are they straightforward conceptually, but proficiency also generally comes quite quickly. Many people prefer others, however.

Relaxation Tapes

Relaxation audiocassette tapes provide soothing sounds, such as the waves of the ocean. Tapes are often a good way to begin practicing relaxation techniques and can also be used before bed to induce sleep. They offer some external stimulation to help you begin to feel calm. If you have no skill at relaxing, this can be a very helpful boost. The down side, however, is that if you continue to use them, you won't learn how to relax the body and mind without listening to the tapes. Since learning to relax on your own is the goal, if used exclusively, the tapes can actually become an impediment to learning how to reduce the symptoms of anxiety.

Physical Relaxation Techniques

There are two major physical relaxation techniques: diaphragmatic breathing and progressive muscular relaxation. Both techniques help treat anxiety in three ways. First, they help you learn how to achieve a relaxed state. Second, they help you to increase your awareness of your physical state so that you can monitor it and learn to stay relaxed when you are anxious in a stressful situation. Third, they provide an alternative focus during an anxiety-provoking situation so that you don't become preoccupied and overwhelmed with the situation and the sensations of anxiety.

Most people who have just begun to learn physical relaxation techniques without tapes practice three to four times a day for ten to fifteen minutes each. They may gradually decrease the amount they practice as they gain proficiency, a process that generally takes some weeks to months, depending on the severity of the anxiety and the consistency of the practice.

In diaphragmatic breathing, you expand your lungs and

breathe primarily by using your diaphragm, the muscle at the bottom of the lung, instead of the walls of your chest. Diaphragmatic breathing will help you to relax your body and slow down your breathing, which is especially useful to combat the hyperventilation that commonly occurs during panic attacks. To assess whether or not you are using your diaphragm when you breathe, place one hand on your abdomen just above the navel and the other on your chest. If you are breathing with your diaphragm, the hand on your abdomen will move first.

To practice diaphragmatic breathing, concentrate on the process of breathing while trying to keep the mind and body as calm and quiet as possible. Sitting quietly and comfortably, silently say to yourself "in . . . out . . . in . . . out" with each breath. Breathe slowly, fully, and smoothly. It is natural for other thoughts to come to mind; simply let them pass without getting you distracted or angry and refocus yourself with the silent repetition of the words. Practice diaphragmatic breathing until you use it unconsciously.

In progressive muscular relaxation, a person slowly clenches and relaxes each of the body's major muscle groups, in sequence, one after the other. The process starts at the toes: first one clenches the toes and then lets them go, then one clenches the ankles and lets them go, then one clenches the calves and lets them go, then the thighs, and so on. Each clenching and unclenching should be gradual and take roughly ten to fifteen seconds.

Unlike the tapes, physical relaxation techniques can be used at any time and in almost any situation. For example, many women use breathing relaxation techniques during childbirth, and people of both sexes use them for visits to the dentist.

Psychological Relaxation Techniques

Beyond physical relaxation is psychological relaxation. The two major psychological relaxation techniques are meditation and self-hypnosis. In classical meditation, one achieves and maintains a sense of calm and physical relaxation by concentrating on a word or phrase while simultaneously letting the body relax deeply. Generally, when people first start meditating, thoughts and images intrude, interrupting the mind's focus on maintaining a sense of calm. Using the repeated word or phrase helps a person maintain a focus on relaxing by overriding any thoughts that do come to mind.

Self-hypnosis can be difficult to learn on one's own and is generally better attempted with someone who is skilled at teaching self-hypnosis. Essentially, however, the technique is to maintain yourself in a comfortable position and imagine that you are in the calmest place possible. It can be on a boat, at the beach, on a mountain, in a field of flowers, etc. You then imagine some appropriate calming and soothing events that occur in that setting, such as waves rolling in, the wind blowing, or birds singing. Try to embroider the scene with many concrete details so that it becomes truly engrossing for you. You then purposely recall this image, and the sense of calm it conveys, in anxiety-provoking situations.

For example, if you are anxious while awaiting a medical procedure, you might think, "I am on an island. I am sitting on the beach near the end of the day. The sound of the foghorn blowing in the distance soothes me. The waves are flowing gently. I look up and see clouds going by. I watch a sailboat slowly going across the horizon. The sand is cool on my feet." As the scene unfolds, you imagine that you are there.

Biofeedback

Biofeedback was discussed earlier and refers to the process by which a person can monitor his body's physical responses through data produced by machines that measure these responses. These machines measure various aspects of a person's physiological state such as the electrical conductivity of the skin, the heart rate, and the types of brain waves produced. These machines were first developed for diagnostic purposes in medicine. For example, brain waves are measured on an electroencephalogram (EEG) in order to diagnose epilepsy.

Some psychologists hook up their patients to these machines in order to provide them with some feedback about how their efforts at relaxing are actually working. After a baseline measurement is taken, a person tries to induce slow breathing, a low heart rate, and alpha brain waves (the type of brain wave associated with a feeling of well-being) in order to induce relaxation and a feeling of well-being. They try various relaxation techniques and use the feedback from the machines to facilitate the process.

A series of six to twelve sessions of biofeedback are commonly employed to help a person learn how to relax. Less complex relaxation techniques, such as the two described above, are practiced in between the sessions to reinforce the learning facilitated by the biofeedback.

PSYCHOTHERAPY

As we have discussed, many people have found psychotherapy an enormously helpful treatment for anxiety. There are many different kinds of psychotherapy available, differing with the philosophy and style of the therapist and the needs and wishes of the patient. Broadly speaking, psychotherapy is a series of meetings between a trained psychotherapist and a client in which they work together to help the client to overcome a psychological problem.

Though a full description of all the different forms of therapy is beyond the limits of this discussion, there are three forms of therapy that can be of enormous help to people with anxiety: behavioral[3], cognitive[4], and psychodynamic[5]. All three therapies can be practiced by therapists in an individual or group setting. Group therapy can be quite powerful but is underutilized in part because many patients resist sharing their problems with strangers.

Behavioral

Behavioral therapy focuses specifically on a person's behavior and seeks to change it through a series of exercises. There are many different behavioral techniques to help a person change behavior. Physical relaxation techniques can be considered a form of behavior therapy. Another type is exposure therapy. There are two main forms of exercises in exposure therapy: *systematic desensitization* and *flooding*. Both require detailed plans developed in conjunction with a psychotherapist.

Systematic desensitization is a process in which the patient and therapist establish a hierarchy of anxiety-provoking situations for the patient, ranging from those that cause no anxiety to those that cause the most anxiety. The patient then practices relaxing in the easiest situation first. When fully comfortable in the initial situation, the patient then progresses to the next situation in the hierarchy, which is slightly harder. A patient practices relaxing at each stage in the hierarchy until the anxiety is mastered before moving to the next stage. Systematic desensitization is a slow process in which anxiety is gradually mastered step by step. If a person becomes overwhelmed at any step, the therapist can scale back the difficulty of each task by breaking it up into smaller increments and increasing the frequency of practice.

Flooding is essentially the opposite sequence. One imagines the most anxiety-provoking situation possible and seeks it out. The experience is purposely overwhelming, especially when it is first begun. However, if a person regularly practices flooding, the other anxiety-provoking experiences in life become much more tolerable. For example, if a person is afraid of open spaces and crowds, he would go to the biggest, most crowded area he could find, such as a mall, on a regular basis. This makes going to the corner grocery seem easy by comparison. Many therapists accompany patients when they first begin flooding and gradually reduce their involvement as the patient gains some proficiency at it.

Cognitive Therapy

Cognition is the mental process of thinking and knowing. Most forms of therapy concentrate on either behavior or emotions, even though almost all rely on a person's cognition and ability to learn in order for the patient to change for the better. In contrast to the focus on behavior or emotions, Aaron Beck, a professor of psychiatry at the University of Pennsylvania School of Medicine, has written many books and articles that examine the cognitive dimension of many psychiatric disorders. In *Anxiety Disorders and Phobias* (1985), Beck acknowledged the multidimensional roots of anxiety disorders but went on to explore the element of cognition in the maintenance of anxiety disorders. He felt that anxiety is maintained by a mistaken or dysfunctional appraisal of a situation. For example, one type of dysfunctional thinking is called "catastrophic thinking," which occurs when anxious people lose their perspective and dwell on the worst possible outcome of any situation and ignore any positive aspects or possibilities. This often occurs in people with generalized anxiety disorder, who think that they have a serious physical illness each time they have an unusual bodily sensation. Although each call to the doctor brings some reassurance that death is not imminent, the next unusual sensation still calls forth the same inappropriate concerns. Over time, people with GAD feel a chronic sense of anxiety about the sensations of their body.

Cognitive therapy is short term, problem oriented, and primarily educational. The cognitive therapist shares his belief that anxiety is due to a faulty appraisal of the anxiety-provoking situation and uses specific techniques to correct a person's distortions. These techniques can include analysis and confrontation of the accuracy of a person's faulty assessment of an anxiety-provoking situation, homework between sessions, and role-playing in the session itself.

Beck gives an example of a young man with social anxiety who wanted to cancel a date because of his anxiety. The therapist and patient set up a specific hypothesis that he could test out: his fear that he wouldn't know what to say. On the actual date, he was less anxious than he predicted, was able to converse, and disproved his hypothesis. Repeated experiences such as these help patients become less anxious in anxiety-provoking situations and function more effectively as a result. This sets up a positive cycle in which increasing success creates strengthened self-confidence and improved functioning.

Cognitive therapy can be enormously useful to help people confront their anxiety and become more active in their own life. It ignores, however, the roots of a person's anxiety, i.e., the traumatic situations that led to the pathological anxiety in the first place.

Psychodynamic Psychotherapy

In this type of therapy, a person seeks to develop some insight and understanding into unconscious thoughts and feelings about people and events that contribute to anxiety. The process involves meeting with a therapist once or twice a week. During the sessions the patient explores both current events as well as events from the past that may contribute to current feelings.

Psychodynamic psychotherapy can be very slow going at first. At least in part, this is because most therapists are reluctant to offer superficial insights during the first two or three sessions because they cannot easily understand all the unconscious thoughts and feelings that play a role in someone's anxiety. Most therapists prefer to wait until they know a patient well before they make interpretations that will meaningfully connect anxiety, current relationships, and some past experiences. For someone who wants some immediate relief, this can be very frustrating.

The regularity of psychodynamic psychotherapy facilitates the observation of subtle manifestations of unconscious feelings. As these previously unconscious feelings become more conscious, the patient is able to acknowledge them, bear them (rather than just repress them), and put them into perspective. Fully acknowledged, these feelings no longer cause "pathological anxiety." We will see how this process works in the next chapter.

Psychodynamic psychotherapy, when practiced by skillful, trained clinicians, can be of enormous benefit. People often learn during a course of this form of therapy that current events and problems in life are directly related to troubling unresolved experiences that they have had in the past. Some people pursue psychodynamic therapy for some months and content themselves with an exploration primarily of current issues. Others want a more complete understanding, which includes a full exploration of issues from the past, and work in therapy for some years.

MEDICATIONS

Several classes of medications can be helpful for people with anxiety. Named for their chemical structure or their physiological effects, these include the tricyclics, monoamine oxidase inhibitors (MAOIs,) selective serotonin re-uptake inhibitors (SSRIs,) beta-blockers, neuroleptics, and buspirone. The decision about whether a patient may benefit from taking any of these medications can sensibly be made only after the full evaluation outlined in the last chapter. The specific benefits and side effects of each medicine need to be considered as well.

Tricyclics

Tricyclics—which include Tofranil, Norpramin, Elavil, Pamelor, Anafranil, and Sinequan—get their name from the three joined rings in their chemical structure. It is believed that tricyclics exert their clinical effects by promoting changes in proteins called receptors in brain cells. The tricyclics abolish panic attacks in about sixty percent of people who experience them. Many people with GAD and PTSD get significant relief from their symptoms of anxiety as well. Anafranil is helpful for people with OCD; Elavil is occasionally used as a sleeping aid because of its tendency to cause fatigue. Sometimes tricyclics produce partial relief with some symptoms of anxiety remaining. Tricyclics are also used to treat depression, childhood bedwetting, attention deficit disorder, and chronic pain. Their effects do not appear to wane over time.

Tricyclics generally take at least two to four weeks to become effective, in part because they are initially prescribed at a low dose and the amount is gradually increased so that the patient can become accustomed to the side effects. Exact dosages vary because of individuals' different rates of metabolism. To make sure the dosage is correct, a blood test may be useful to determine the exact level of a particular tricyclic in the body.

Many people find the day-to-day side effects of dry mouth, light-headedness due to low blood pressure, constipation, sweating, blurry vision, weight gain, and fatigue significantly troubling, which has limited their popularity. Tricyclics do not have any apparent long-term side effects.

MAOI Inhibitors

Monoamine oxidase inhibitors, or MAOIs—which include Nardil, Parnate, and Marplan—get their name because of their effects in the body: They inhibit the breakdown of a class of substances called monoamines, which includes neurotransmitters like adrenaline. This action increases the amount of adrenaline in the brain, which many researchers believe accounts for their clinical effects. MAOIs are helpful in treating patients with panic attacks, PTSD, and some people with severe anxiety that falls under the category of anxiety disorder, not otherwise specified. MAOIs are also commonly used in the treatment of depression.

Although MAOIs can be very effective, many patients do not like to take them—and many physicians do not like to prescribe them—because of the possibility that they can cause a stroke. Ingestion of substances that are similar to adrenaline or that can be used in the synthesis of adrenaline can cause sudden high blood pressure, which can lead to a stroke. One common such substance is tyramine, which is present in a number of foods such as aged cheese, sour cream, yogurt, processed meats, broad beans, liver, chocolate, bananas, pickles, sauerkraut, licorice, beer, and wine. Patients must avoid these foods while taking MAOIs. Additionally, MAOI users need to avoid all medicines that contain substances that are commonly found in cold remedies, such as antihistamines like Benadryl, decongestants like Sudafed, and narcotics like Demerol, codeine, and Percodan. MAOIs also have other side effects, including dry mouth, light-headedness, weight gain, inhibition of sexual functioning, jitteriness, and insomnia. MAOIs also take two to four weeks to become effective because they must be started at a low dose and the amount slowly raised.

Selective Serotonin Re-uptake Inhibitors

SSRIs—which include Prozac, Zoloft, Luvox, and Paxil—get their name from their effect in the body: They inhibit the ability of a neuron to recapture, or re-uptake, the neurotransmitter serotonin. As we discussed in chapter 4, neurotransmitters such as serotonin are chemical messengers sent by one neuron to another across the space between them, called the synapse. By limiting re-uptake, more serotonin remains to affect the postsynaptic neuron. This effectively increases the amount of serotonin in the brain, which supposedly accounts for the clinical effects of these drugs. SSRIs are usually prescribed for depression but are sometimes helpful for people who have panic disorder, agoraphobia, GAD, PTSD, OCD, and anxiety disorder, not otherwise specified. Like tricyclics and MAOIs, SSRIs also take two to four weeks to work.

SSRIs became quite popular shortly after their release in the mideighties. This was due in part to their minimal effects on blood pressure, which made them especially useful for elderly patients.

Additionally, some people with chronic depression felt that they improved in a truly remarkable way, an effect that was described in the book *Listening to Prozac* by psychiatrist Peter Kramer. However, many people notice a diminution in sexual desire and difficulty with their sexual response, and a small percentage of people experience agitation.

Beta-blockers

Beta-blockers—which include Inderal, Corgard, and Tenormin—get their name because they block the action of adrenaline on beta receptors, a protein in some nerve cells. Since many of the symptoms of anxiety appear to mimic those of an adrenaline surge, many researchers have hoped that these drugs could provide significant benefit to people who suffer from anxiety. Some people get some relief from the symptoms of anxiety preceding such situations as presenting a lecture or taking a test. Daily use of beta-blockers, though helpful to lower blood pressure, is generally ineffective for anxiety.

Neuroleptics

Neuroleptic medications such as Thorazine, Risperdal, Trilafon, and Stelazine (trifluoperazine) are generally used for more severe psychotic symptoms such as delusions and hallucinations. These medications are sometimes useful, however, for people whose anxiety is so overwhelming that it disorganizes their thinking. Unfortunately, if used regularly for longer than one year, neuroleptics can have irreversible side effects such as tardive dyskinesia, a condition in which a person experiences uncontrollable lip smacking, and hand and body muscle movements. They also cause unpleasant day-to-day sensations such as restlessness, sedation, muscle stiffness, and emotional and cognitive blunting, which some people describe as feeling like a zombie. These side effects limit their usefulness for the vast majority of people with anxiety.

Buspirone

BuSpar (buspirone) is chemically distinct from the other agents listed above and is useful for some people with anxiety. Although it can take several weeks to work, it is not addictive, and people do not become tolerant of its beneficial effects. It tends to be used primarily for GAD. Many people, however, do not find it particularly effective.

All of these drugs can be useful in the treatment of anxiety, but even this brief description of them demonstrates why many physicians and patients think first of benzodiazepines for relief of anxiety: All these other medications have problems, too. Tricyclics, MAOIs, SSRIs, and BuSpar all take two to four weeks to work and their effectiveness is by no means certain. Beta-blockers don't really work at all, and neuroleptics have many unpleasant day-to-day side effects and potentially irreversible ones with extended use. It is highly unfortunate that all too many people see medications as the primary mode of treatment for anxiety. Although drugs can seem like an easy and sensible solution, the relief of chronic anxiety should rely primarily on relaxation techniques and psychotherapy, with medication used primarily as a supplement.

This brief description of relaxation techniques, psychotherapies, and medications serves only to highlight reasonable alternatives to benzodiazepines, not as a comprehensive assessment of their value. As I noted at the start of the chapter, only a patient and psychiatrist working together can make an appropriate decision about which treatments to use to address the problems identified in the initial evaluation. In the next chapter, we will see how these treatments can be used to help a person eliminate a dependency on benzodiazepines, master anxiety, and move on in life.

· 10 ·

STOPPING BENZOS AND TAKING CHARGE

To stop taking benzodiazepines is a process with a number of different stages. People take different amounts of time to get through each stage because of differences in dosage, duration of use, type of anxiety, duration of anxiety, and a host of other individual factors. Some steps typically go very smoothly, while others tend to be more difficult. Work on some stages will occur during work on other stages. I have helped hundreds of people go through the process of getting off these drugs and know that although each person may take a somewhat different path, anyone who is willing to keep on trying will ultimately be successful.

The real goal, however, is not just to get you off the benzodiazepines, but also to help you stop being the victim of anxiety. Although I've seen some people stop the drugs on their own, few of them learned other ways of managing anxiety. Some stumbled into other unproductive ways of managing their anxiety, such as using other drugs, becoming overly dependent on other people, or maintaining a markedly constricted life, but as a result they continued to allow anxiety to control their lives. To fully accomplish the overall goal of learning to master your anxiety, you will need additional help beyond just stopping benzodiazepines, and I strongly recommend that you work with a psychiatrist who is prepared to get to know you and can help you through this difficult process. I have outlined the stages of recovery, but only you and your psychiatrist can plan and carry out a program that takes your individual needs into account.

Because the best way to understand how to accomplish the task of getting off benzodiazepines and mastering anxiety is to observe how other people do it, I will describe how the patients I introduced earlier regained control of their lives. Each person had a unique experience of anxiety and dependency and brought different skills, strengths, and weaknesses to the effort, and each of them went through the different stages in his or her own way. Your experience is unique as well, and you will need to forge your own path through these stages. I will describe the issues relevant to each stage in the next chapter so that you can apply them to yourself. For now, let's look briefly at what those stages are.

1. MAKING A COMMITMENT TO STOP

When people who are dependent on benzodiazepines come to see me, I describe the drugs' dangers and drawbacks. After hearing my piece, a few people storm out of my office, muttering epithets or calling me names. The vast majority, however, hear me out politely. Of those, probably one in three leave my office with no intention of ever seeing me again or acknowledging any of the ideas that I have tried to explain. These people have no intention of stopping their usage.

Most people who consult me about benzodiazepine use and anxiety know that their lives are not going well but are astonished to hear that their use of medications is one of the reasons. Though skeptical, they are willing to make a serious attempt to stop their usage. I know that if they make the initial commitment to work with me, their progress will resolve their doubts.

A small portion of people agree with what they hear. They are pleased to meet somebody who wants to work with them in getting off the medications. These people are often able to stop their usage without any difficulty and are grateful to accomplish that. The finding that some people are able to stop without significant difficulties has been noted by others.[1]

Making a commitment to stop can be difficult and scary because it means breaking the familiar habit of taking a pill and replacing it with other unknown and untried methods. Most people find it reassuring when they find out that they should taper their dosage slowly and not stop all at once, and that they will have a

chance to learn some new methods before they give up their pills
for good.

Sometimes people do not make the internal commitment to
stop benzodiazepines and go along with my recommendations
only because other people want them to, or because they are afraid
I'll be mad at them. This is a situation similar to an attempt to lose
weight in order to please a spouse rather than to please oneself.
Unfortunately, superficial compliance usually gives way to full-
scale resistance at some point.

A genuine internal commitment to stop benzodiazepines differentiates itself from passive compliance when obstacles such as increased anxiety or decreased satisfaction with people or events in
life emerge during the tapering process. People who have made the
internal commitment strengthen their resolve to meet the challenge and overcome it. People who are passively complying with a
doctor's plan find almost any obstacle too much for them, and
they quickly bail out.

People who passively comply with recommendations often
hope that a psychiatrist can "fix" their anxiety the way an orthopedic surgeon fixes a broken leg. Pathological anxiety is not a broken
leg, however, and psychiatrists are not like surgeons who can fix
things. Psychiatrists *can* help patients learn to use some powerful
tools to help them in their struggle with anxiety, but patients need
to do the work themselves.

Hard or easy, making the internal commitment to stop benzos
is the most important step in the whole process. Without it,
chronic use and chronic anxiety drive a person further and further
into an unsatisfying shell of a life. Once the commitment has been
made, however, the path to a satisfying and meaningful life can
begin.

2. HANDLING THE PHYSICAL SENSATIONS OF ANXIETY

Intensified symptoms of anxiety will occur when the dose of benzodiazepines is even minimally reduced, and most people need
some specific aid to help them when this happens—most commonly, relaxation techniques and medication.

3. TAPERING YOUR DOSAGE

Usage is tapered slowly, gradually, after some skill has been developed in managing the symptoms of anxiety.

4. DEVELOPING ALTERNATIVE METHODS TO MANAGE ANXIETY

In this phase, people choose practical and satisfying long-term strategies that interest them and fit their particular personality in order to reclaim their lives from anxiety.

5. CONFRONTING THE SOURCES OF YOUR ANXIETY

Gradually coming to terms with thoughts and feelings about current and past events is a hard, but essential, step in the process of becoming free from the control of anxiety.

6. MAKING PROGRESS

When people make the effort to try and improve, they do get better! They experience less anxiety and learn to handle stressful situations more effectively.

7. TAKING CHARGE

As people give up these drugs and learn to manage anxiety effectively, they feel good about themselves and confident about their abilities. They feel that they are back in charge of their lives and are no longer controlled by anxiety.

Susan

As we have discussed, Susan had begun experiencing panic attacks with no obvious relation to any particular experience in her life except going to a restaurant. She had quickly become dependent on Ativan, and even though she saw a couple of psychiatrists and therapists over the next few years, she stayed on the Ativan. She continued to experience anxiety but felt that it didn't particularly interfere with her functioning. By the time she came to see me about her flying phobia, however, she realized that anxiety was getting in the way of the life she wanted. Susan was receptive to the idea of living her life without being controlled by anxiety, even though it would be hard work for her.

I explained that she would need to learn and practice relaxation techniques, and Susan quickly understood their importance and agreed to begin to practice breathing techniques and meditation. I recommended that she also engage in systematic desensitization, in which she would practice getting on a plane even before she was scheduled to fly. Sometimes people with phobias join groups of other people with similar phobias, but Susan declined to become involved in a group, stating that she didn't want to talk about her problems in front of strangers. I also recommended weekly sessions of psychotherapy not only to help her through the tapering process but also to identify the sources of her anxiety and resolve them more satisfactorily than she had before. Susan was somewhat leery about giving up the Ativan. When I explained how it sabotaged her efforts to feel better, however, she agreed to go along with my recommendation that we slowly taper it. We agreed that tapering would start only when she had learned how to manage the symptoms of anxiety more effectively.

Because she needed to get a handle on anxiety right away so that she could start to fly and accept the promotion, Susan decided to go on other medications. She agreed on a trial of imipramine, a tricyclic that is effective in substantially reducing the intensity and frequency of panic attacks in many people. Additionally, I prescribed Inderal to help minimize her symptoms of anxiety as much as possible when she actually traveled by plane. Although neither of us liked the idea of Susan using three medications simultaneously, it made the most sense in view of her need for rapid improvement. Our goal was to gradually get her off all three.

Susan accepted the promotion. She practiced the relaxation techniques religiously and quickly became proficient in putting herself in a state of calm. Imipramine made Susan's mouth dry, but after a month on it she noticed fewer panic attacks. From two or three a week, the frequency dropped to one. One week she had none. She also began to notice that she was less worried about panic attacks.

To help her with her fear of flying, we set up a hierarchy of anxiety-provoking situations related to the flying experience. The hierarchy consisted of twelve stages ranging from imagining herself in the airport and on a plane to actually getting on that plane. On the first day, she twice spent fifteen minutes imagining going to the airport terminal and waiting in line. On the next three days, she spent one minute imagining getting to the terminal and waiting in line, and the rest of the two periods imagining boarding the plane. In sessions over the next four days, she focused on sitting in the plane. Several days were spent focusing on the takeoff, flying, and landing of the plane. Throughout the imaging practice sessions, she used the breathing technique to keep herself calm. She always performed the exercises in a comfortable chair in her bedroom, an image that she hoped would evoke a calming feeling when she was actually flying.

Three weeks before her first scheduled flight, she went to the airport, the next step in the hierarchy. She was anxious in the terminal but was able to maintain a sense of control with her breathing techniques and the knowledge that she wasn't flying on a plane that day. Two days later she went again. Two weeks before her flight she went a third time and explained her fear to one of the airline personnel. She was allowed to enter a plane that had just landed and was being cleaned. Susan thought that it would be hard for her to enter the enclosed space of the plane, and indeed it was. She had to stand in the boarding area for a few minutes, concentrating on staying calm by using the meditation technique of repeating *ocean,* the word that she had chosen as her mantra. She pushed herself to enter the plane but stayed close to the door for several minutes. Initially, she sat in a seat in the first row from which she could see the door. She brought out a mystery novel that she was in the middle of and began reading. It was hard for her to concentrate on the book, but her goal at this time was just to tolerate staying on the plane. She kept telling herself that she could get off anytime she wanted to. After fifteen minutes she began to feel a little bit more relaxed. She realized that even though she could get off at any time, she had now been on so long that she obviously didn't need to get off. She moved to a seat in the middle of the plane. As she stayed on the plane, she gradually became even calmer. Additionally, she began to feel a growing confidence that she would be able to get on the plane in two weeks. The airline flight attendant came by at this point and told her she would need to leave. She kept up her imagery work and made two more trips to the airport before her first flight.

On the day she was actually scheduled to fly, Susan went to the airport three hours ahead of her scheduled departure. She was anxious but hoped that she would again experience the feeling of confidence that she had felt during her practice sessions. She took her usual dose of Ativan. Although she had brought along some extras, she didn't take them. She carried the Inderal with her and planned to take it an hour before flight time so that it would be in her system when she had to get on the plane. She spent part of the next two hours reading and part meditating. She admitted to me later that she also spent part of this time worrying, because it seemed like a big moment in her life. She would have to give up the job if she couldn't fly but would likely advance even further in the company if she could. An hour before flight time she took the Inderal. She had hoped that she wouldn't need to but then decided that she would take advantage of every aid that she could. She asked the airline boarding staff if she could get on board early so that she could take her time and get on the plane slowly. She repeated the steps that she had taken when she went on the plane before. She felt anxious—very anxious—but with the aid of her meditation techniques, the anxiety didn't escalate to the point of a full-blown panic attack. The flight was two hours long, and as it progressed, Susan became slowly calmer and was even able to read. She became slightly more anxious as the plane landed and taxied to the terminal. As she got off, however, her anxiety quickly receded. She continued to be somewhat anxious for the next couple of flights. Each time she flew, however, she became more confident and less anxious. She stopped the Inderal after only three flights.

After Susan flew successfully a few times, we set up a schedule for her to taper her Ativan. As she had always varied her dose depending on how anxious she felt or thought she was going to feel, we set up a tapering schedule to begin at 2 milligrams a day, the lowest dose that she usually took. She was quite hopeful that she would be able to accomplish the taper without significant difficulty. Although she did experience a mild increase of anxiety with each dosage reduction, she had no major problems.

During the three months when Susan worked successfully to overcome her fear of flying and begin the tapering of the Ativan, we continued to meet in weekly psychotherapy. She accurately perceived her quick progress in experiencing fewer panic attacks, but she also described a side of herself that wasn't confident, that felt unsure and worried even when she wasn't having a panic attack.

We then began to explore the sources of Susan's anxiety. She said that her mother had suffered panic attacks, too, causing her mother to be somewhat isolated and constricted while Susan was growing up. She said she really did not want to be like her mother and had never wanted to face this side of herself.

I asked her what it was like to grow up with her mother being so constricted. At first Susan described her mother rather blandly. I pressed her to recall any specific activities she had engaged in with her mother outside the home, but she could remember none. Susan said that her mother was often supportive of her in the things that she was doing in school but found it very difficult to leave the house to cheer her on in person. In fact, while growing up Susan missed many activities that would have required her parents' help. For example, she'd never learned how to swim because no one had ever taken her to a swimming pool or given her swimming lessons. She had never played any kind of organized sports while growing up, and although this was partly because there were not as many sports available for girls as there were for boys, it was also because she could not stay after school for sports or other activities because her mother could not pick her up.

Susan did remember wanting very much to play in the school band. Although she did take some clarinet lessons—there was a clarinet teacher available at school—she wasn't able to practice very much at home. Her mother apparently needed "quiet" at home in order to manage her own anxiety. After a short time the clarinet lessons stopped because of her mother's frequent requests that Susan not play. Susan now realized that this period of time coincided with one of her parents' separations. Her mother had simply been too overwhelmed with her own problems to pay attention to Susan's desires.

After sympathizing with Susan about the fact that she had not been able to do a number of things that she had wanted to do growing up, I asked her if there were things she currently wished to do but wasn't doing. She was surprised at the question because she had always thought of herself as a strong person who knew her mind and got what she wanted. After remembering all that she didn't get growing up, however, and remembering her feelings of frustration and anger, she realized that she often experienced those feelings in her current life—especially with Kevin, her current boyfriend. She realized that she had difficulty asserting herself in her relationship with him, and that this had been true in her relationships with other men in the past, including Mark, her first serious boyfriend.

Initially Susan had liked Mark at least partly because nothing seemed to bother him and he seemed able to feel confident in any situation. She now realized, however, that she had used his confidence to bolster her own. She became aware that the feelings of anxiety, unsureness, and lack of confidence that she still felt at times had a long history. She realized that she had experienced feelings of insecurity and anxiety even before she had met Mark. She had always thought the panic attacks, which began after she met him, were the first time that she had ever felt anxious.

As our sessions continued, Susan began to be aware that although there were many things that she liked about her current relationship with Kevin, there were some things that she didn't like. At times he drank and went out without her. At those times she felt that she couldn't "reach him" and felt quite distant and separate from him. Kevin didn't seem to understand that whenever he drank, his behavior changed in a manner that Susan didn't like, or that she didn't like the fact that he sometimes stayed out drinking with his friends all night. He would never really say where he went, and she felt somewhat uncomfortable asking him. The next day he was usually hung over. Susan realized that she had always downplayed the amount that Kevin drank and had minimized the fact that she didn't like it; she also came to the realization that one of the reasons that she didn't like Kevin's drinking was that it reminded her of her father. Although her father rarely drank, he was often absent because of his extramarital affairs and the separations from her mother. Although she had always loved her father and he had been kind to her, she felt a painful absence whenever he wasn't around. Kevin's unavailability when drinking reminded her of her father's absence.

Susan now realized that she had always had some mixed feelings about Kevin. Although she liked the fact that he seemed to be "in control," in fact her relationship with Kevin made her anxious. She realized she was anxious about being involved in a relationship with somebody who drank so much. She realized that she was somewhat fearful of getting involved in a close relationship with anybody because of her own parents' experience.

She also realized that she had never learned how to address her anxieties in a way so that she could fully resolve them. Thus when she was having doubts about Kevin, she had no way to manage them. Nobody in her family had talked openly about personal difficulties. More important, however, nobody in her family had helped Susan overcome obstacles in a positive and successful manner. Every time anyone in her family had met an obstacle or a difficulty, they had retreated—her father into extramarital affairs, her mother into reclusiveness.

After six months of work with me, Susan knew that, contrary to her original belief, a number of factors had contributed to the onset of her anxiety attacks: her ambivalence about her relationship with Mark, which had continued in her relationship with Kevin for many of the same reasons; and her own long-standing inability to manage her anxiety in any way other than trying to bury it—the style of helplessness that she had learned from her family's response to obstacles. In addition, Susan and I both felt that there was probably a biological component to her anxiety because of her mother's history of panic attacks and her own experience of intense anxiety and its appearance early in her life.

Susan knew there was very little she could do about the biological aspect of her anxiety. She realized, however, she did not have to remain helpless in the face of new challenges. She also realized that she still wanted to try playing the clarinet. She rented one and began taking lessons. She grew increasingly dissatisfied in her relationship with Kevin, finally broke up with him, and began going out with other men.

Susan soon recognized that when she started seeing anyone, it was difficult for her to trust her own feelings. When she brought up her inability to be clear about her feelings for an engineer with whom she had gone out a few times, she realized that she was feeling ambivalent because the man drank and because he was somewhat domineering. This realization occurred after about a year of therapy and many months after she had stopped any use of Ativan.

Susan now became frustrated because she began to feel that I was not providing enough direction for her, that I was too quiet and didn't talk enough. She wanted direction about what to do in her relationship with the engineer. She felt that I was withholding my opinion of what she should do. I responded by asking Susan if she felt incapable of sorting out her own feelings and developing some strategies of her own. Susan acknowledged that she did. I asked her if this feeling of helplessness was one that was familiar to her from the past. Susan acknowledged that, like anybody else, she had felt frustrated at times but had not known what to do about it. Acknowledging that I had not given Susan significant amounts of advice, I asked her if her current feelings were similar to ones that she experienced with her mother: namely, that when Susan felt helpless growing up, she had looked to her mother for help, her mother hadn't given it, and Susan had felt angry and frustrated. Susan remembered when she had been unable to figure out a way to get to the clarinet lessons and had finally given them up. She had felt quite angry at her mother because her mother hadn't helped her figure out a way to get to the lessons. She realized for the first time that she had often wanted other people, in this case, myself, to tell her what to do.

This session was very important for Susan because she became fully aware for the first time how her parents' inadequate support for her contributed to her anxiety and lack of confidence as an adult and how she still hoped that someone would make things better for her. She grew tearful when she realized that she was hoping for something that she would never get—a supportive adult who could help her know what she should do. Although she was preoccupied with her sadness over the next several weeks, she also realized that, as an adult, she no longer needed someone to direct her. She possessed all the skills that she needed in order to resolve frustrating situations for herself. For instance, she was quite capable of discerning her feelings about the engineer and did not need me or anybody else to tell her what to do about them. What she lacked was not advice from other people but the belief that her feelings were reasonable and the confidence to act on them. Susan continued in therapy for another six months. We continued to focus on her feelings about her parents and those that arose from their divorce. As we continued our work, she gradually reduced her imipramine without difficulty. Her panic attacks did not return.

We began to wind down the frequency of our sessions after about two years. Susan continued to be anxious about her ability to make a sensible choice about marriage and said that she would probably need to see me if she began seriously to consider marrying someone. In fact, however, I received a letter from her about a year later stating that she was engaged and felt confident that the man was the right choice for her.

Jim

Jim came to see me after he became tearful in his internist's office because of worsening anxiety. He was clearly caught in the syndrome of the Benzo Blues. He was anxious almost all the time, leading to irritability with his family, and he had difficulty functioning at work even though he had been taking Klonopin for two years.

He told me right way that he hadn't wanted to come to see a psychiatrist because he had always been able to solve any problems by himself. When I asked what had led him to change his mind, he admitted that his internist refused to prescribe any more Klonopin, and he felt that he couldn't get along without it. I asked him how it felt to depend on the Klonopin. He admitted that he disliked using any drug because it made him feel as if he were defective, but he thought that the Klonopin was the only thing standing between him and a nervous breakdown. I told him that I could understand that he didn't want to see a psychiatrist—no sensible person does, especially people who are used to taking care of their own needs. I also told him that I wanted to help him to regain his self-sufficiency. He warmed up a little at this point. He admitted that he was so angry at himself for having such difficulty functioning that he was taking his anger out on me in the same way that he took it out on everyone around him in the rest of his life.

Jim was primarily conscious of his difficulties at work. As it is for many men, his ability to perform as the breadwinner was central to his self-esteem. But lurking behind his difficulties at work were a number of feelings that arose because of his father's untimely death when Jim was eight. Jim was aware of the role that his father's death had played in his life. He had always believed that he had coped as well as possible, and he had promised himself to be there for his children. Consequently, it was a surprise to him, and a disappointment, that he was having difficulty being the loving father he wanted to be. We agreed that both work and home would need to be addressed in our sessions together.

Jim's initial hostility to me arose because he was frustrated and embarrassed: He wanted to be doing much better in his life. Once we had broken through his combativeness, it was clear that he was very motivated to try almost anything in order to feel better and get his life back on track. He quickly understood that he needed to find some new ways to manage his anxiety, and he readily agreed to learn and practice the progressive muscular relaxation technique. He also agreed to meet with me every other week for ten sessions, a compromise between my recommendation for a more open-ended treatment and his wish for monthly sessions in which we would only monitor his progress.

Jim was nervous about stopping his 4 milligrams of Klonopin a day but understood that its continued use was keeping him from getting better. We set up a tapering schedule. Jim insisted that he wanted to drop his intake down to 3 milligrams a day immediately, reduce it to 2 milligrams in one month, to 1 milligram in two months, and stop the Klonopin entirely in three months time. This was faster than I recommended, but he was not dissuaded by my concern that such a rapid pace might lead him to increase his dose if he became overwhelmed.

Jim soon decided to speed the process even more. When I saw him two weeks later, he announced that he had stopped taking his Klonopin entirely. He had decreased the dose every three days in order to avoid having a seizure and had taken his last dose the night before. He acknowledged that he was very anxious but was sure that he could handle his anxiety, since he knew that the intensity of his symptoms was due to physical withdrawal. He said that he felt more effective at work and was starting to socialize again with his friends. He said that he had practiced the relaxation techniques but told me that they were ineffective. He vowed to keep practicing, however.

Jim was so intent on getting better as fast as possible that he was jeopardizing the chance that he would get better at all. I cautioned him about trying to go too fast, but he brushed aside my concern, saying he was already more confident at work and less irritable at home, in spite of increased anxiety. He left the session with the plan to buy several books about early childhood development so that he could learn how to feel more comfortable as a parent.

Unfortunately, Jim's optimism was short-lived. His wife called me a few days later and said that he hadn't been able to sleep for two nights and had even taken a sick day from work. When she put him on the line, he was somewhat embarrassed, but I assured him that trying too hard was nothing to be ashamed about. My main concern was to help him follow a plan that was more realistic than simply stopping his Klonopin and hoping that his enthusiasm would be sufficient to change his life. He agreed to go back on 3 milligrams a day and to follow our original schedule.

When we next met, he had restarted his Klonopin and felt much calmer. He acknowledged that he had underestimated the difficulties and realized that he needed to become proficient at relaxing himself and slowing himself down. Besides the progressive muscular relaxation technique, I also recommended that he practice the meditation relaxation technique.

He was already feeling more comfortable at work, but I knew that the real source of his anxiety, his capacity to function effectively as a father, needed to be addressed as well. I recommended that he proceed with his plan to read books about infants and children.

When he next came in, he told me that he had purchased a whole series of children's development books, each of which explored the development of a year of a child's life. He had already read the first three and expressed surprise at the emotional complexity of the lives of infants and toddlers. Over the next month he continued his reading, ending up with the book on nine-year-olds. He was quite somber as he related his growing awareness that his father's death had not just left him angry and determined to be a "better father than him." He now realized that he'd never had a chance to share any ongoing activities, such as sports, with his father. He didn't remember laughing with his father or even if his father had a sense of humor. He didn't remember ever hugging his father.

He said that he now realized why he felt uncomfortable with his children. He knew only how to perform the concrete tasks of fatherhood; he had no idea of how to enjoy the day-to-day interactions that fathers have with their children. He decided for himself that he had to learn how to feel comfortable with his children, how to play with them, how to touch them, and how to relax with them. He had talked openly with his wife about his difficulty feeling comfortable with their children and had begun to watch very closely as she interacted with them. He also arranged some play-dates with other fathers and their children and talked with them about what they did with their children.

Jim had no difficulty tapering the Klonopin at the rate we had initially agreed on. He found that he enjoyed the peacefulness of the meditation technique and continued to practice it daily even after he had stopped the Klonopin. He became less anxious as he grew more aware of his feelings about his father's death and began to be more comfortable with his children. He realized he would be a good father as long as he was able to be involved with his children emotionally, even if he wasn't able to give them all the material things he wanted. His anxiety about work lessened because he no longer felt so tense about his home life. He found he was able to concentrate more effectively at work, which allowed him to finish his work on time and resume his lunch-hour contact with his friends.

Jim's treatment lasted only five months, a shorter period of time than I had initially anticipated. He was able to accomplish a lot in that short period, however, because his motivation was quite strong. It is unfortunate that benzodiazepines can misdirect a person's energy so subtly that even someone with such strong motivation to do the right thing can become tangled up. Confronting the unhealthy role played by benzodiazepines can allow a strongly motivated person to improve quickly.

Janet

As with Jim, when Janet came in to see me, I thought that treatment would be long and arduous—and as it happened, this time I was right. Though many doctors and patients feel that someone over seventy shouldn't be expected to engage in intensive treatment, age alone shouldn't be the deciding factor. I refused to believe that Janet was a lost cause because I have known too many people in their seventies, eighties, and even nineties who lead vibrant lives. I knew that she could feel a lot better, too, and live for many more years being in control of her life. I hoped her spryness and sense of humor would prove helpful during our work.

Luckily, Janet readily saw that she needed some help. She understood my concern that Serax was contributing to her difficulties and agreed to a gradual taper, even though she wasn't sure how she would tolerate being without it. She knew that her anxiety and depression were becoming worse, and said she was willing to "follow all the doctor's orders." I was troubled by her words because they implied that the treatment would be my plan for her, not our plan together. I hoped that some initial success might transform Janet's compliance into a strong internal commitment. I agreed to prescribe Paxil for her depression, and she agreed to try relaxation tapes and practice relaxation breathing. I stressed the importance of her developing other methods of coping with anxiety. My attempts to bridge the difference in outlook about how she was to improve, whether through my recommendations or through her efforts, were initially successful, at least superficially.

Within four weeks Janet was feeling calmer and less depressed, and we started to taper the Serax. She had been taking 10 milligrams two or three times a day, and we agreed that for the first month she would restrict herself to only two times a day. As alternative methods of managing her anxiety, she agreed to begin taking a daily walk and going to the library once a week to choose books to read. When feeling acutely anxious she planned to take a bath while listening to music. Additionally, she planned to prepare some videotapes that she could watch to distract herself when she was anxious.

Over the course of the first month, Janet found it difficult to restrain herself from taking the third daily dose. The next month I gave her only sixty tablets—enough for two a day but no more. During this time I got a call from her internist, Dr. Crandal, who told me that Janet had called him to ask for a prescription renewal of Serax. I thanked him for not prescribing any more so that she wouldn't have two doctors prescribing different medications for the same problem.

When I called Janet on the phone, she was a little embarrassed about calling Dr. Crandal, but she also expressed some anger at me. She said that she had taken the third dose of Serax a few times because she couldn't get along without it. She felt that I didn't understand how desperate she felt when she got anxious. When I questioned her more closely about the times that she had taken the third dose, I learned that they had occurred when she wasn't seeing any of her family. Either she was unoccupied or plans that had been made had fallen through. She acknowledged that she had a very difficult time being alone, and she also admitted that she hadn't been regularly practicing her relaxation techniques. I reminded her about the importance of developing some other ways of managing her anxiety so that she would have some options for herself. She had been to the library a couple of times but hadn't begun taking a daily walk, hadn't prepared any videotapes, and hadn't tried taking a bath while listening to music. I could tell that she was mad at me, but she reluctantly agreed to pursue these methods of managing her anxiety and refrain from increasing her Serax dose.

By the next time we met, Janet had started walking and was practicing the breathing techniques. She admitted it was hard for her to put her needs first and engage in any activity in which the goal was to improve her own life, not someone else's. She said this was just the way she was. I asked her if there was ever a time when she had wanted something for herself and didn't get it. With visible irritation she answered that of course there were things that she didn't get in life, just like anybody else. When I asked her to tell me about one, however, she was able to say only that nobody's life was perfect. She became somewhat tearful but kept her composure.

Clearly, my question evoked some powerful feelings in her, and these feelings interfered with her ability to carry out the program we had outlined. I could see that we would need to uncover some of those feelings in order to remove the resistance. I decided to change the usual order of the stages of treatment, which I outlined earlier in this chapter, and begin to uncover the sources of her anxiety at once.

I pressed Janet further to tell me about some of her unmet wishes in life. She told me that she wished that she had been able to have a garden when she was growing up—she would have liked the peacefulness of a garden, the satisfaction of growing plants, the beauty of flowers—but there was always so much to do. As an adult she visited gardens in museums and parks and watched television shows about different kinds of flowers and gardens. She said she had always wanted to visit Zen gardens in Japan.

As I listened, I could see that she obviously knew a great deal about horticulture. Taking advantage of her offer to "follow doctor's orders," I asked her to take out a couple of books about the subject from the library, with the plan of designing a garden herself. My hope was to strengthen her wishes so that she would be more motivated to try to satisfy them, and to see if I could find a way to help her talk about her feelings. She gave me an angry look but also smiled and said that she would.

By the time she next came in, Janet had designed not one garden but three. She described in detail how they would look during different seasons, the amounts of shade and light each would need, and the amount of work that would be necessary for upkeep. When I asked her which one she might have liked best when she was growing up, she said that she would have chosen the smallest of the three; she had had so much else to do while she was growing up that she need to minimize any additional work for herself. When I asked her what she had done, she began to open up about all the tasks that fell to her when her mother went to work: laundry, cleaning, cooking, and supervising the younger children. She described one particularly vivid memory when two of her younger brothers played with matches in a closet and almost burned the house down. She had been outside hanging up the wash. The boys had taken off in the other direction when the fire started, so Janet didn't realize what was happening until a neighbor saw smoke and called the fire department. Luckily, the fire was extinguished soon enough so that there was little damage to the house. Her parents weren't angry at her; they knew that it wasn't her fault. But Janet felt that it was. She never felt confident after that because she never knew what might happen next. She constantly felt guilty and scared and became more vigilant in watching the other children. She felt that she could never take her eyes off them lest something terrible happen.

As Janet talked about the fire and her feelings, she became more animated than I had yet seen her—more alive, more upset, but somehow more present in the room with me. I could see that she had dropped her guard a little. She could sense that, too, and she began to put it back up. She finished her description rather quickly with the statement that everyone probably had problems like hers. Not wanting to get into an argument with her, I agreed that many people had painful experiences growing up. I added that people also handled them in different ways.

When she didn't come in for her next appointment, I learned that Janet was back in the hospital with colitis; she had become dehydrated and needed intravenous feeding. I called her in the hospital to hear from her how she was doing and expressed my hope that she would improve quickly. She was released in several days. When she next came in, she told me that she didn't want to talk about anything "upsetting" because she needed to focus her energy on "feeling good." I asked her to tell me how long it usually took for her to recuperate from a bout of colitis, and we spent the rest of the session talking about her experiences of previous exacerbations of the illness, how debilitated she felt, how depressed she would feel being stuck in bed, and how she would perk up as soon as she was able to get around again. She insisted that she be allowed to take three Serax a day, and I agreed that her impaired medical condition made a reduction in dose inadvisable. By the next week, she was feeling a little bit better.

In the next few weeks we talked more about gardens and more about Janet's experiences in caring for her siblings. She began to see that besides the worry that some disaster would befall them, she also had other feelings. She enjoyed their successes. She was proud that she was able to care for them in her mother's absence. The more we talked about those times, however, the more she began to acknowledge her frustration that she had not pursued anything for herself. It was hard for her to articulate what, as a child, those things might have been because she had shut them off so completely in order to take over her mother's role, but she could see that identifying her own needs and wishes was difficult for her.

At my prompting, Janet admitted that it was reasonable for her to focus on improving her psychological health, just as she had focused on her physical health following the hospitalization. She agreed to practice relaxation techniques more consistently and to taper her Serax. I was far more hopeful that she would be able to be successful in our work together because it was clear that her commitment now came from inside her; she was no longer just following my "orders."

Over the next several months Janet was gradually able to reduce and stop the Serax. We continued to meet and discussed other experiences while at the same time working to develop a more satisfying balance between meeting her own needs and those of her family. We discussed not only her assumption of her mother's role but also her maintenance of a caretaking role in the family when she became older and her siblings became ill and then had their own children. She began to see that although it may have been necessary for her to help out initially, it was her own decision to stay in the caretaking role. She was even able to acknowledge her regret about avoiding marriage and not having her own children.

As we began to come to an understanding of how she came to be so anxious in her later years, Janet volunteered less frequently to help out with her family. She was still quite involved, but more on her terms than on theirs. Her calls to Dr. Crandal grew less frequent, and her bouts of colitis decreased in intensity and frequency as well. She saw for herself that strong feelings about issues in her life would lead to an exacerbation of her colitis, and she began to use those incidents as a signal that something was bothering her. Her family was pleased to see that she was feeling less anxious and seemed to understand that she needed to set some limits about what she would or wouldn't do.

Janet came in with a particularly hardened case of Benzo Blues because of the length of time that she had spent avoiding her feelings, the years of inconclusive medical tests and misinformed explanations of her difficulties by Dr. Crandal and herself, the exacerbations of a medical problem caused when she became anxious, and her personality style of ignoring her own emotional needs to the point that she could barely follow through with treatment. These difficulties required some modification to the order of the stages that were needed in her treatment, but they did not prove insurmountable. Janet's own motivation and willingness to keep trying, even when she was angry with me, helped her succeed. As Janet and those who cared about her could see, it's never too late to change.

Marilyn

When Marilyn had been living with her daughter and her family for a year and a half, Jeremy, her eldest son, came to visit. Because he lived on the other side of the country, he and Marilyn had not seen each other for almost two years. He felt Marilyn was doing badly, and he was concerned because he felt that she was addicted to Xanax and Dalmane. Although Marilyn denied that she was addicted, she did acknowledge that she "depended on them." Having abused alcohol in the past, her son had some experience in Alcoholics Anonymous, and he knew that Marilyn's use of benzodiazepines and the problems in her life were linked. When he insisted that she see a psychiatrist who could help her try to get off the medication, she agreed to a consultation with me.

When Marilyn first came in to see me, she acknowledged that she was having a difficult time. She told me about the death of her husband, her gradual slide into anxiety and use of Xanax and Dalmane, and her increasing difficulty with day-to-day functioning. She discussed her feelings of depression and her use of Prozac. Although she felt that the Prozac helped her to feel less depressed, she disliked its side effects of insomnia and increased anxiety. She mentioned the death of her mother and former reliance on her father and husband in passing, but she clearly saw little connection between her current distress and her experience early in life.

I spent most of the first session developing a shared understanding of how difficult Marilyn's recent experiences were and how overwhelmed she felt. As we were reaching the end of the session she asked me how I would help her. I explained that her treatment would involve one hour-long session of psychotherapy weekly to help her focus on her feelings and learn more effective ways of coping with them besides holding them in and depending on others to care for her. I also explained that we would first help her with the concrete issues of managing anxiety and then look at the sources of her anxiety. Marilyn understood that there would be some overlap between the two aspects of treatment. She would first need to learn and practice relaxation techniques. We then discussed the usefulness of the Prozac and agreed that switching to an antidepressant that didn't cause insomnia and anxiety would be sensible.

Knowing that Marilyn felt that Xanax was helpful for her, I spent some time explaining how I felt it was interfering with her life. I described the Benzo Blues and pointed out that her dependency had contributed to her isolation, anxiety, depression, and her gradual withdrawal from the activities in her life that she had found meaningful in the past. I explained the problem of physical dependency on benzodiazepines, of which she was only minimally aware. I also told her that although she was unsatisfied with her life, she had little chance at present of improving her life because she was not involved in things that would bring her satisfaction. I told her I could help her, but that it would take hard work.

Marilyn was clearly troubled at my belief that Xanax was making things worse not better for her; she said that Xanax was the only thing that helped her. My response was to question her closely about how useful it really was for her. She acknowledged that the relief from Xanax was temporary and that her symptoms of anxiety kept recurring. She also acknowledged that when the anxiety did return, she felt her only option was to take another Xanax. She defended herself quickly; she didn't take a large dose, she said, nor did she take more than what her internist prescribed.

"I'm not an addict," she insisted. When I agreed with her, and she could see that I brought up her use of Xanax because of my genuine concern for her well-being and not because I was criticizing or blaming her, she confessed that she didn't really like to take it. "The problem is that I'm scared to be without it. I wouldn't know what to do with myself when I get anxious if I didn't have it."

Marilyn was reassured when I told her that I would help her to learn to manage her anxiety before we started to taper the Xanax, and that we would taper it very slowly. I explained that we would first change her Prozac to a low dose of Pamelor, a tricyclic antidepressant that often causes mild sedation, which improves sleep, and that she would spend a month or two learning and practicing relaxation techniques including breathing exercises. We agreed that she would go to a nearby bookstore and purchase a couple of relaxation tapes to counteract her concern that she wouldn't be able to tolerate sitting quietly at first. She understood that she needed to practice other techniques as well, and she agreed to work on breathing exercises while listening to the tapes in preparation for practice without the tapes.

When Marilyn left the session she said that she was glad that she had come in and expressed some hope that her anxiety, and her life, would improve. When she came in the next week, however, she stated that although she had tried to practice the relaxation techniques, they didn't work. In fact, she became more anxious whenever she tried them. I explained again that relaxation techniques are always ineffective at the outset; only after extensive practice do people notice their benefit. I urged Marilyn to continue to practice for twenty minutes, four times a day.

She had stopped her Prozac and started on the Pamelor. She

said she noticed that she was able to fall asleep more easily but hadn't noticed any change in her anxiety during the day. I explained that it takes many weeks to eliminate Prozac from the body and that it can take some weeks for the Pamelor to become effective. We agreed that she would increase her dosage of Pamelor up to 100 milligrams each day.

The next week Marilyn reported that although she was able to practice the relaxation techniques, she could do so only with the aid of the tapes. Although she saw this in a negative light, I pointed out to her that she had in fact made some progress because until now she hadn't been able to relax at all except with the Xanax. I not only encouraged Marilyn to keep using the tapes in order to improve her ability to relax herself but also emphasized that she needed to begin to practice the breathing exercises that we had discussed earlier.

By the fifth session, Marilyn acknowledged that she felt less anxious after she practiced a breathing technique. She slept better and felt that the agitation caused by the Prozac had faded away. She also felt that her baseline mood was unchanged. She did not feel more depressed, always a possibility when changing antidepressants.

We discussed a schedule to taper her Xanax, which Marilyn had been taking at a dose of 0.5 milligram three times a day. She was scared because she had not been without Xanax for some years. She felt that she absolutely needed to have the pills. I agreed that her concern was reasonable, and we agreed that she would reduce her dosage by a quarter of a milligram a month, which would mean that she would be off it in six months. After that she would go off the Dalmane, too. I emphasized that she should not try to accelerate the agreed-upon tapering schedule.

At our next appointment, Marilyn reported that she had decreased the Xanax for two days as agreed but then felt so anxious that she was unable to bear it and went back to her original dose. I once again emphasized the importance of getting off the Xanax if she wanted to develop a more satisfying life for herself. I noted the progress that she had made in using the relaxation techniques successfully. She agreed with all I was saying but said, "I'm scared." Nevertheless, she agreed to try the reduced dosage again for the next month.

Marilyn was more anxious for the next few weeks. She diligently used her relaxation techniques, however, and was justifiably proud of her ability to remain on the lowered dose. "Jeremy has been pleased with how I've been doing, too. He's been calling almost every week. He was glad that you told me I should come off the Xanax."

After about two weeks on the lowered dose, the anxiety appeared to lessen a little bit. Marilyn understood that her body was gradually adjusting to the new dose. Over the next couple of months the tapering went as scheduled. During this time Marilyn and I worked on helping her to develop new ways of managing her anxiety. We both knew it would be important for her to have a reasonable range of methods that would help her develop different ways of coping with different levels of anxiety, which would insure that she could always use one if another weren't possible. She decided to work on four new methods: exercising by taking a brisk walk, reading a book, working on needlepoint, and talking with either family members or friends.

Over the next few months, Marilyn found it most helpful to talk with her family members and friends when she felt especially anxious. She explained to them that she wasn't looking for advice, and that it wasn't their job to make her feel better; however, if they would listen to her talk about her concerns, it would ease her mind. Her daughter was often able to talk, but when she wasn't, Marilyn sometimes called one of her sons. All three were glad that she was finally beginning to come out of her shell.

Marilyn also found that a brisk walk was a helpful activity. Not only did she get out of her daughter's house, but she also felt that the stimulation from being outdoors often led her to think about something other than her own concerns, such as environmental issues, the role of humans in the physical world, and the beauty inherent in nature. She also began to take an interest in improving her physical health, something to which she had never paid much attention before.

Although she hadn't been able to concentrate enough to enjoy needlepoint or reading for the previous few years, Marilyn made an effort to take up these activities again. She sometimes found it hard to concentrate when she was anxious, but a few minutes of relaxing breathing usually calmed her down enough so that she could stay engaged for an hour or two.

When Marilyn came in after three months of the tapering, however, she said that the next couple of weeks were likely to be extremely difficult because her daughter and her family were going on vacation and Marilyn would be alone in the house. She didn't think she could manage being on her own if she tried to decrease her Xanax. I pointed out that we had anticipated that there would be times that would be more difficult than others, but that it was necessary to forge ahead nonetheless. I also pointed out that this was an opportunity for Marilyn to use the other activities to manage her anxiety.

While her daughter was away, Marilyn had no source of transportation for herself. Although it took some effort, she twice went shopping at a nearby market to buy food. On one of her trips she met a friend she hadn't seen for some time who invited Marilyn over to her house. Marilyn surprised herself by agreeing to go. She learned that her friend had become involved in a weekly quilting group. Although Marilyn knew very little about quilting, she had always been interested in it and agreed to join the group. Because she had no transportation of her own, her friend offered to pick her up. Over the next few months Marilyn continued to attend meetings of the quilting group.

She made some important progress as a result of developing other methods of managing her anxiety. Not only was she finding anxiety less troubling to manage, but many of the activities she took up to manage it also led her to become more involved in parts of life that she had neglected. She gave herself opportunities that had not existed for her before. Marilyn could see for herself the progress that she was making, that she was beginning to take charge of her life.

We now began to talk more specifically about some of the anxiety-provoking issues in Marilyn's life. We discussed what it was like for her to be the director in her own life and not always relying on other people. She admitted that she was scared of being alone. At first she talked mostly about how she had depended on her husband and her father to make decisions for her, but as our sessions continued she began to speak more directly about the loneliness she had felt years earlier when her mother had died. She felt that she had lost the one person who could have helped her to make a place for herself in the world as a woman, wife, and mother. This period of psychotherapy was very painful for Marilyn because she still had deep feelings about her mother and her mother's death that were painful to unearth. She increasingly came to realize that her mother's death had continued to shape how she approached life as an adult forty years later.

Marilyn was now down to a dose of only 0.25 milligram of Xanax twice daily. In the month that followed she reapplied for her driver's license. She didn't like to impose on other members of the quilting group for rides, nor did she want to give up the group.

Marilyn had continued to go to church during the past few years but had stopped being involved in any of the church's activities. She now decided that she would volunteer two mornings a week at the hospital where her minister served as chaplain. She found that the work she liked best was transporting patients within the hospital because it gave her a chance to talk to people. Marilyn felt that she was able to make the patients' time at the hospital a little nicer, and she increased her time to four days a week.

By the time the final month of the tapering came, Marilyn was to take one pill during the day, but only if she felt she needed it. During that month she did take one Xanax on several days but on most days did not. Increasingly she realized that when she felt the urge to take the Xanax, it was because she was feeling anxious about a situation in her life that she felt unable to solve. Now that she had proved to herself that she could solve some of her problems, however, she felt increasingly confident that she could solve other issues that arose—without taking Xanax.

The next month when she saw me, Marilyn asked if she could keep a few pills around "just in case I need them." I told her that I didn't recommend this, that she would then be carrying around the temptation to continue to feel like a victim and feel incapable. I pointed out that since Marilyn was no longer taking Xanax, she was clearly over the physical addiction. However, I cautioned her that she would likely continue to feel a psychological addiction for some months to come. We agreed she would stop the Dalmane now as well. Although she experienced a few sleepless nights, probably due to physical withdrawal, overall she finished the tapering process without significant difficulty.

Once Marilyn was off the Xanax, she felt that it was safe to drive again, and she began to get out more. It turned out that she had a flair for quilting. A nearby store agreed to take on her work to sell it on consignment. Marilyn's minister also asked her if she would help organize the church's benefit for sick children, and she readily agreed. She was able to enlist some quilting friends. One of the people in that group invited a friend who had recently become a widower. On the day of the benefit this man appeared to be paying as much attention to Marilyn's quilt sales as to his own booth. At the end of the day he asked her if she would join him for coffee at a nearby restaurant. Although Marilyn didn't know him very well and wasn't even sure that she liked him, he seemed nice and she figured, "Well, what do I have to lose?" As it happened, he had a good sense of humor and was fun to be with. Although she had previously felt that she had no intention of going out with anybody ever again, much less getting married, over the next several months Marilyn did begin to see this friend regularly.

By the end of our therapy, Marilyn felt that she was doing well. Her children agreed and were glad to see that she was more confident and social. Marilyn's daughter noticed that she went to her medical doctor less frequently and felt that Marilyn was more confident than she had ever been when her husband was alive.

She decided to try going off the Pamelor because she didn't want to be dependent on any medication. Tapering the Pamelor took some months but occurred without any difficulty. Marilyn stopped seeing me shortly after that, after we had met for about two years. She continued to go out with her friend and was considering marrying him when we last met. She was also considering going to college to obtain an associate's degree in business for possible work in accounting. She told me that she had given up her dream to go to college as a teenager, but now it didn't seem impossible anymore. Although she wasn't able to afford her own apartment when we parted, she hoped to at some point in the future.

Debbie

Debbie's anxiety was fairly severe. She had been anxious all her life, and when she first came to see me because of agoraphobia, she hadn't left her house in two months. She had been skeptical about meeting with me because she wasn't sure what I could do to help her. I told her she would probably always have more anxiety than most other people but that we could certainly help her to lead a life that was less limited by her anxiety and more satisfying to her. I also told her it would take some work on her part. She groaned and humorously rolled her eyes but said she knew her treatment wasn't going to be easy.

Debbie could see that her use of Librium wasn't helping, and she readily agreed to taper and discontinue it over a four-month period. She and I both felt that her first task would be to gradually go out of the house more and more. We set up a schedule in which each day she went out farther and farther from her house for longer and longer periods of time. To help her accomplish this, Debbie practiced progressive muscular relaxation techniques. Even though she had never had a panic attack, she wanted to try a medication to help her feel less anxious and, after a discussion about possibilities, decided on a trial of Prozac.

At first, it was uncomfortable for her to push herself even to get out the door, but she gradually made progress. She felt less anxious and more confident on the Prozac. She found some part-time work folding inserts for the local newspaper, a job that required little contact with others but did get her out of the house.

From the start of our work, Debbie was able to talk about her anxiety fairly easily with me. She described how it had impacted her life growing up and how it had been intensified by her parents' drinking. It was hard for her, however, to feel comfortable around other people. I suggested that she consider group therapy to feel more comfortable sharing her thoughts and feelings with other people and learning a bit about what makes them tick.

Debbie initially refused even to consider group therapy. As we talked more about it, however, she could see that it made sense to her, and that her negative reaction was based on her pattern of avoiding anything that might make her anxious. She decided to meet with a therapist who ran groups for people with anxiety and agreed to a trial of twelve sessions in one of her groups. She and I also agreed that we would continue to work together during this time.

Debbie was surprised to find that she actually liked the group. The eight other members were friendly and continually cracked jokes, referring to themselves as the "scared bunny group," talking openly about the different things that led them to be anxious, and discussing some of the things, both productive and unproductive, they did to manage their anxiety. Each of the members continued to struggle with anxiety and the limitations it caused in their lives. Some were on medication, two on benzodiazepines. Several others experienced agoraphobia, and Debbie felt an immediate bond of sympathy with them. One man had abused alcohol in the past, which made her uncomfortable because of her experiences with her father. As the weeks progressed, Debbie became an active member of the group, sharing her own experiences and joining the discussion of other people's. Not only did she feel less alone in battling her anxiety, but she also was able to take advantage of some of the strategies that other group members used to feel more comfortable in the outside world. In time she left her job at the newspaper and began working full-time in a large bookstore. Although she had to interact with a lot of customers there, she did so in a very friendly atmosphere and felt quite comfortable after an initial period of mild anxiety.

Over time, Debbie gradually became more irritated at Andy, the man in her group who drank alcohol. Though he was nice at times, he sometimes made statements that were just plain mean. It turned out that his alcohol use wasn't just in the past; Debbie smelled liquor on him during one of the meetings. She didn't confront him during that group meeting, but she talked about it with me the next day when we met for our individual session. She was angry that he had lied, pretending everything was okay during the group. She was reminded of her father's distortions about his drinking habits and his verbally abusive behavior in front of her friends.

At the next group meeting, Debbie confronted Andy about his drinking. She told him that she didn't like his mean statements about other people, didn't like his drinking or lies, and felt that he was being disrespectful to the rest of the group with his behavior. She also said that he was shortchanging himself if he was going to sabotage his own treatment by drinking and lying. She had never confronted anyone as strongly as she did Andy. He was somewhat taken back, she reported to me later, but apologized for coming to the previous meeting after he had been drinking. Other group members agreed with her statements and complimented Debbie for having had the courage to speak what was on their minds as well.

The confrontation with Andy proved to be somewhat of a breakthrough for Debbie. She found that although she had been scared to confront him, she knew she was right, and she knew that she would have the support of other members of the group. She realized that she had often felt afraid of expressing her anger and began to be more aware of other people and situations in life that led her to be angry. She told her father about her anger at him for his past drinking and abusive behavior. He had stopped drinking years before and had already acknowledged to Debbie how his behavior had hurt other people, but this was the first time she had openly expressed her anger toward him.

In short order, Debbie decided that she was doing well enough to get off Prozac, and she stopped it without difficulty. We stopped our work together, but she decided that she wanted to continue in her group. When we last met she had started going out with one of her co-workers at the bookstore, her first serious relationship.

Many people with agoraphobia, and other anxiety disorders as well, derive enormous benefit from simultaneous group and individual psychotherapy, although third-party payers may not like to pay for both treatments and some patients don't want to put in the effort. Group and individual therapy can augment each other quite nicely, especially when the individual therapist helps a person to process upsetting reactions to other group members and to develop new ways of relating to other people, first in the group and then in the outside world.

Tom

Tom had coped with social phobia quite productively at times in his life: He had learned some meditation and relaxation techniques and used them successfully in the past. He had attended assertiveness training seminars, which he had found somewhat helpful. He quickly accepted my assessment that although there was probably a biological component to his anxiety, he had become mired in an unsatisfying relationship and work situation because he relied on Tranxene to make things better rather than dealing with those problems directly. He also knew that although anxiety was temporarily getting the best of him, he could get back in control again.

After our first meeting, Tom started practicing his relaxation techniques again, and we set up a tapering schedule for his Tranxene. He had no difficulty getting off the drug. He could see that he needed to end the unsatisfying relationship with his girlfriend and within a short period did so. It turned out that she was prepared to end the relationship as well because she felt that it was going nowhere.

It was harder for Tom to be more assertive at work. We both knew that his father's verbal abuse contributed to Tom's difficulty asserting himself, but he couldn't see exactly how. As we explored some of the incidents of his father's abuse in detail, he began to see that he had habitually buried his anger at his father. He was especially angry at having been thrown into the swimming pool in front of his friends. Tom had never expressed his anger at his father directly because he knew that his father would merely ridicule him again. He realized that he held himself back when he became angry with people because he was afraid it would all spill out at once. His apparent passivity was really a way to manage intense anger.

With this realization, Tom knew that he needed to learn how to be more assertive in an appropriate way. He began to prepare for minor confrontations with customers and his boss at work by rehearsing what he would say. He became more confident of his ability to be more assertive when he could see that he could confront an unpleasant situation successfully. We stopped our work together after about five months.

Tom's treatment was relatively brief because he had managed his anxiety successfully in the past, regressing when an overbearing boss who bore a striking resemblance to his father came his way and retreating into taking Tranxene. Once he realized that he could do better without taking medication, he was motivated to address his anxieties and problems more directly. With the work in psychotherapy that explored his repressed anger at his father, he uncovered and resolved one of the sources of his anxiety. He knew he would probably always be more anxious in social situations than most other people, but his anxiety no longer interfered with his ability to function.

Sam

Sam had had so much treatment over the years because of PTSD from the Vietnam War that it was difficult for him to commit himself to learning a new way to manage his anxiety besides taking the Valium. When I framed the treatment as a challenge that I hoped he could meet successfully rather than as an order that he had to follow, however, he could see that I wasn't trying to control him and he grew more cooperative.

Sam's first move was to give up drinking his eight to ten cups of coffee each day. Although he was distinctly tired for the first two weeks or so and had moderately severe headaches, he also recognized that he was less anxious. He didn't want to try any other medications, but I urged him to try Desyrel to help with sleep because he still awoke with nightmares. After a couple of weeks on the Desyrel he found that he did sleep better, and he decided to continue taking it. Positive though these changes were, however, they weren't sufficient to help him because of the severe intensity of his anxiety from PTSD.

I spent some time explaining to him that relaxation techniques would help him to relax, but first he needed to learn *how* to be relaxed. I referred him to a local psychologist who helped him develop the ability to relax with the help of biofeedback. Sam then continued to practice both breathing and progressive muscular relaxation techniques. My experience with other veterans has shown me that many need vigorous physical activity as an outlet for their anxiety and high energy level, so I recommended karate as an alternative strategy to help him when he was feeling anxious. He could practice daily in his basement and whenever he felt especially anxious or upset. We both felt that more passive activities such as reading were unlikely to be effective for him.

Sam continued with his group therapy, deriving considerable comfort from contact with other veterans with similar experiences. The group, the cessation in caffeine, the regular practice of relaxation techniques, the improvement in sleep from the Desyrel, and his practice of karate were sufficient to reduce his anxiety enough so that he was able to get off the Valium. We both knew that no treatment would erase the emotional scars, anxiety, and bitterness from his time in the war, but he didn't need to compound his problem with a dependency on drugs.

Betsy

When I first saw Betsy, the music teacher, for evaluation of her difficulties arising from the development of PTSD after a fire, it was unclear to me how much she would be able to improve. She had been reluctant to meet with a psychiatrist just after the fire and had hoped to be able to overcome her problems by herself. She had been badly scared by her experience more than a year before but had received Klonopin as her only treatment. Consequently, she had spent a year with ongoing anxiety, poor sleep with nightmares of fires, fearfulness, and no help integrating the experience and her feelings in any useful way. When it became obvious to her that she wasn't coping well, and when her principal suggested that she come to see me, she agreed to come in.

I was concerned that during the year without treatment, in order to manage her feelings Betsy might have developed some counterproductive coping mechanisms that would now be hard for her to change. Fortunately, however, Betsy had managed her distress primarily by retreating from activities related to teaching students at the school and by taking the Klonopin. She hadn't used other drugs, developed any medical problems, or begun to rely excessively on others. She still enjoyed some of her usual activities of observing the national political scene by reading papers and magazines and watching television, seeing her family and friends, playing the piano and violin, and listening to music in many different forms: classical, musicals, opera, and country music. However, she suffered from low self-esteem because she believed that she should have been able to shake off her anxiety by now and get on with her life.

Betsy understood my explanation about the problems resulting from continued use of Klonopin, and we set up a tapering schedule to begin in one month. She agreed to a trial of Pamelor to help her to feel less anxious and to improve her ability to sleep. She agreed to practice breathing techniques and exercise daily by both walking and swimming. Because she had also become much more negative than she used to be and had difficulty finding pleasure in her life, I suggested that she investigate and study a new area of music that she knew little about. She agreed and decided rather playfully that she would practice the drums, saying that since little old ladies never play the drums, maybe it would shake her up and get her moving.

Over the first month of treatment her sleep and anxiety improved. Betsy felt that the Pamelor helped her to sleep with many fewer nightmares and less anxiety during the day. She then began to taper the Klonopin.

She informed the school's principal that she planned to continue teaching when school started back up in September. This gave us only a month to help Betsy feel more confident about being in the building itself. We set up a program during which she gradually spent more and more time at the school, first in another teacher's classroom and then in the music room. She decided to bring her drum set down to the school so that she would have something to do while she was there.

Throughout the summer we met weekly so that Betsy could talk over the experience of the fire and her reaction to it. It was difficult for her to open up at first, in part because she had spent the last year holding in all her emotions. Once she did open up, however, her feelings came tumbling out. During the fire she had been afraid for her life, of course, and then relieved at escaping. She was proud that she had acted decisively enough to break the window when there was no other route of escape. She felt lucky to still be alive, and she appreciated the wonderful gift that life is. Mostly, however, she was angry. She was furious at Michael, the janitor, for handling his cigar carelessly. Smoking was prohibited at that school, but the authorities had ignored Michael and his cigars—because he had been a fixture there for many years, because everyone liked him, because he had always done a good job, and because he smoked only after school hours. But he still shouldn't have been smoking, and the principal shouldn't have let him do so. She was also furious at the school board because the building's sprinkler system wasn't sufficient. The school building had been neglected for years, and the administration of the school could never seem to find money to maintain and upgrade it appropriately. Following the fire, everyone had apologized to her and Michael no longer smoked, but the sprinkler system still hadn't been upgraded. Their carelessness could have ended her life, Betsy said in both anger and tears.

She had never told anyone how angry she was because she didn't want to seem critical of the school to which she had devoted many years of her life. Once she had opened up her feelings, however, she could see that she was still afraid when she went back to the school because it was still unsafe. She decided to write a letter to the principal and the school board to request that they address the sprinkler system. She expected that they would take her letter seriously, because she knew that they thought highly of her. The principal immediately had the system inspected. Although the system technically met the standards required by law, several deficiencies were highlighted. At the urging of the principal, the school board authorized a complete overhaul so that the alarm and sprinkler system would be more effective in the future. Additionally, two fire extinguishers were placed on opposite sides of every room so that fire would not prevent access to one of them, as had happened to Betsy.

She was grateful for the response of the school administration. Although she knew that she would never forget the fire, her feelings, and the initial lack of response by the administration, her fearfulness receded, and she began the school year confident that things would go smoothly.

They did. Betsy was able to teach after school without excessive anxiety and got along well with Michael. She tapered off the Klonopin without difficulty. She decided that she didn't like the drums (too loud!) and stopped playing them, but she had enjoyed her brief time with them. She decided that she would stay on the Pamelor for a while because she was worried about having nightmares of fires and waking up in a sweat. We stopped meeting for therapy, but I continued to see her a few times a year to evaluate the usefulness of the Pamelor. She tried to get off it a couple of times, but the nightmares returned each time. She finally decided that she would stay on it indefinitely.

Betsy became more anxious each year in late May, the anniversary of the fire, but was able to make it through without changing what she was doing. Although she stayed on the Pamelor and continued to feel somewhat anxious when she saw stories about fires on the television or in the newspapers, she continued to function well.

Peter

Peter, the engineer who struggled with OCD, knew that he would probably experience his obsessions and compulsions for the rest of his life. He was aware that recent research into the brains of people with OCD has strongly suggested that the disorder is primarily a biological illness, even though the symptoms may first appear during a period of stress.

The severity of Peter's symptoms had led him to become dependent on Ativan, and he used a very high dose—from 6 to 8 milligrams a day. He didn't like taking the drug because of the effects on his memory and the diminished muscular coordination that he feared might impair his driving. Besides taking clomipramine, a tricyclic medication that has been proven to help many people with OCD, he knew of no other methods to help himself, however, and so he stayed on Ativan for years. He came to me requesting that I help him to get off it. He also hoped to become more socially outgoing and successful at work.

I could see Peter's intense distress. We discussed the importance of practicing relaxation techniques, and he agreed to integrate these into his life. I referred him to a behavioral psychologist, who used biofeedback to help strengthen his ability to induce relaxation. The psychologist also taught him other psychological techniques to help obsessions and compulsions. Peter found two of the techniques especially helpful. The first one allowed him to schedule brief periods during the day when he was to give free rein to his tendency to worry excessively, permitting a greater feeling of freedom from those urges in the intervening times. The second technique was to snap an elastic band around his wrist as an alternative to handwashing.

We obtained a blood level of his clomipramine and raised the dose when it came back below the therapeutic range. Although he felt that the higher dose was more beneficial, it significantly diminished his sexual drive and impaired his ability to have an orgasm. He decided that he wanted to try Luvox and Prozac, two other medications with demonstrated usefulness in the treatment of OCD, to see if they could provide any improvement in his symptoms without causing sexual dysfunction. Prozac didn't help his symptoms at all. Luvox was somewhat better. It helped his compulsions substantially, although it had little effect on his obsessions. Higher doses of Luvox caused the same sexual dysfunction as did clomipramine, but lower doses did not. Peter raised and lowered the dose, depending on whether he was more troubled at the time by his compulsive symptoms or the sexual dysfunction that higher doses caused.

Peter and I set up a schedule for tapering his Ativan. He wanted to proceed fairly rapidly because he disliked the side effects, and we agreed that he would decrease by 0.5 milligram every two weeks. I told him that a slower taper might be somewhat easier for him, but he was determined to proceed as quickly as possible. Although his anxiety definitely worsened during the months of the tapering, he was able to maintain the schedule that we had set up.

Several months after Peter stopped taking the Ativan, he felt a little better. His obsessions and compulsions were no worse, and they were under even better control when he could tolerate a high dose of the Luvox. Once he was off the Ativan, he no longer experienced memory impairment, and he felt more confident about his ability to drive. He began making some efforts at establishing social contacts with others. He joined a church and attended their monthly dances. He began to date women from his church and job. He had always performed well in his work as an engineer and had hoped that he could rise to a managerial position; however, he decided that this was unrealistic for him, given his discomfort around other people. He began to devote some time and energy instead to learning more about computers in the hope that he could develop a sideline in some aspect of the burgeoning "information superhighway."

It is unfortunate that this was the best we could do for Peter. Current treatments for OCD are inadequate, although there is hope that recent technological advances in brain imaging will enhance our understanding of the illness and lead to more effective treatments in the future.

Heather

Heather's difficulties were not confined merely to anxiety and a dependency on Xanax. Her experience of parental divorce, sexual abuse by her father, and intermittent abuse of alcohol, and her difficulties in establishing any semblance of a satisfactory intimate relationship led her to feel emotionally overwhelmed with feelings of emptiness, loneliness, and low self-esteem on a daily basis. Fortunately, Heather also had some considerable strengths on which to build: She was smart and held a successful job as an attorney and so could afford extensive treatment.

The first stage was for her to learn some coping skills to manage her feelings of emptiness more productively than using drugs, sex, or work. She agreed to stop drinking and go to Alcoholics Anonymous meetings several days a week. She quickly grasped the role that alcohol was playing in her life: It provided daily soothing, but left her internal feelings unchanged. She understood the importance of staying off all alcohol and realized that her use of Xanax was merely a substitute.

Heather also agreed to a tapering schedule for the Xanax. We both felt that the Zoloft was as helpful as any antidepressant was likely to be, and so she stayed on the same dose of 150 milligrams.

Heather tried many different relaxation techniques. She found tapes and the breathing technique helpful. She also learned self-hypnosis, which she found most useful of all. For alternative anxiety-reduction strategies, she began exercising at a health club, reading fiction, and taking luxurious baths.

We met for hour-long sessions twice a week to establish each of these aspects to her treatment and monitor her progress. She had no real difficulty understanding the rationale for each of the treatments and was strongly motivated to use them. She was able to get off the Xanax without too much difficulty.

Heather's real problem was that as a result of the sexual abuse, she always felt on an emotional roller coaster. Each time we talked about some aspect of the abuse, other memories and thoughts would be stirred up as well. As a result, the first year of her treatment was fairly tumultuous. She became acutely suicidal when her father came to town on a surprise visit, and she was briefly hospitalized. Although she no longer blotted out the memories of the abuse with drugs or alcohol, she wasn't yet ready to confront her father with how angry, sad, and devastated the abuse had left her. She decided not to see him at all and told him over the phone that she was thinking about the past and couldn't see him for the present. He apologized for the abuse, but she felt that his apology was just his way of manipulating her again, this time to obtain forgiveness rather than sexual favors.

Following the hospitalization, Heather joined a therapy group for adult women who had been sexually abused as children, which she found enormously helpful. Not only was she able to discuss the experience and her feelings with other women—something she had never done with anyone except me—but the other group members had many suggestions for handling various aspects of their life as adults that she found helpful. For example, some of the women had confronted their abusers and suggested that Heather wait to do so until she was further along in her treatment. They also suggested that she avoid any sexual relationships with men for the time being because the reminders of her experience with her father would contaminate the new relationship too much. Their suggestions confirmed her own sense of what she should do.

Over the course of the next several years Heather and I continued to meet twice weekly, and she continued in the group as well. She established a new repertoire of ways to manage the aftereffects from the sexual abuse. Rather than run from her feelings any way she could, she would bring them up with me and the group to understand where they came from, how they had evolved in the years since the abuse, and how to manage them productively. She finally confronted her father and decided she would have little to do with him because he seemed only superficially repentant. She began dating again but proceeded very gradually with any sexual activity so that she could enjoy it without being overwhelmed. She decided that she would stay in the relatively nonadversarial area of estate planning in her work at the law firm. Although it was not as interesting as she would have liked, estate planning was something she was good at, provided a very healthy income, and rarely led to emotionally painful situations.

The support group for sexually abused women eventually disbanded as members finished their own work and drifted away, and Heather and I gradually reduced the frequency of our sessions to once a month. She didn't want to meet less frequently, however, because there continued to be situations that reminded her of the abuse and she felt that our sessions helped her to stay anchored. Like many victims of sexual abuse, she continued to experience an elevated level of anxiety that required ongoing work to minimize. She continued on Zoloft because it helped her periodic depressions.

As we have seen, though the road out of the Benzo Blues has some basic features, it varies tremendously depending on the individual characteristics of the person, the specific anxiety disorder that he or she has, and any problems in a person's life. Your experience of the Benzo Blues and what will be helpful for you will not necessarily duplicate that of any of the people I've just described. In the next chapter we'll look at how some of the treatments that they used can be helpful for you.

· 11 ·

OUTLINING YOUR PROGRAM FOR STOPPING BENZOS

It is essential to your overall recovery that you work with a psychiatrist who can help you to navigate the process of detoxification. Although some people try to "go it alone" or decide to quit benzodiazepines just by getting decreasing doses from their primary care doctor, they run the risk of failing by not getting treatment for anxiety and the underlying sources that cause it. You and your psychiatrist will develop your own plan together, which, as we've discussed will likely include the following steps.

1. MAKING THE COMMITMENT TO STOP

Though you may want to get off benzodiazepines or be worried about the dangers of not getting off them, you may have mixed feelings about stopping them as well. You may be worried because you know it will be a difficult process. You may feel that the medication helps you to feel calmer, but at the same time you may want to be free from depending on it so that you can live a life in which you, not your anxiety, are in control.

Doubts about the wisdom of getting off may merely gnaw at you at times, and they may scream at you at others. Like Janet, you may struggle with taking the necessary steps in the early stages because of your doubts. It's important to recognize that these doubts are not the sensible voice of reason, however, but the desperate voice of the drugs pleading with you to keep taking them, keep taking the easy road, and keep letting anxiety rule your life.

The most important step of all, therefore, is the first one: the commitment you make to yourself that you will stop your usage, even if you do have doubts and even if it is a hard task. As you will soon find, progress usually begins quite rapidly.

It can be very helpful to enlist family members and friends to aid you as you follow your program. They can't make you less anxious, but they can support your desire to stop these drugs, provide encouragement when you feel discouraged, and give you feedback about your progress. I often meet with family members or friends of the patient to clarify the overall goal and anticipate some potential trouble spots during which support for the patient can be helpful. I also clarify that it is not the role of family members or friends to take anxiety away or perform everyday functions for the patient.

2. HANDLING THE PHYSICAL SENSATIONS OF ANXIETY

You will experience physical symptoms of withdrawal and symptoms of anxiety when you first decrease your usual dose. As you know only too well, these symptoms are exceedingly unpleasant and very difficult to tolerate, and are probably an important reason why you are still taking your pills. The second step, then, is to manage the physical sensations of anxiety before the dose is decreased.

It is essential that you learn and practice the relaxation techniques I described in the last chapters. You should try several different methods to see which work best for you. Practicing three to four times a day for fifteen to twenty minutes each time generally begins to help after a few weeks, although you may need some months to notice substantial benefit. Unfortunately, there is no shortcut to this step. If you do not notice rapid benefits—and many people with severe anxiety do not—try increasing the frequency of your practice up to four to six times a day and the duration up to twenty minutes each time. As your sense of relaxation improves, the frequency and duration can decrease. Keep a daily diary of your practice, recording each session and rating your anxiety on a scale of one to ten when you are finished.

There are three essential elements for success in practicing relaxation techniques. First, when you begin to practice, you need to be as calm as possible and in quiet surroundings, so you can focus on the act of relaxation itself and not on the situation that is troubling to you. To accomplish this, you need to schedule time for yourself each day away from other people and activities. Many people set up a weekly schedule to ensure that they will get the practice that they will need.

Second, you will probably find that you become even more anxious when you begin to practice relaxation techniques. This is common and, more to the point, normal. Anxiety is often lessened during activity. It stands to reason that when you don't have any activity to take your mind off what is making you anxious, you will experience more anxiety. It is important to slog through this period and continue practicing the relaxation techniques regularly. Nobody is good at these exercises right away.

Third, you must practice faithfully. In the same way that a tennis player must practice each day in order to have a backhand that will work during a big match, you need to practice relaxation techniques each day so that you can calm yourself reliably in situations that would normally lead you to be anxious.

The use of relaxation techniques alone may be insufficient to manage the symptoms of withdrawal that occur when you first start to taper the benzodiazepine. Another way to mange the physical sensations of anxiety and withdrawal is to use the other medications described in the last chapter. Whether this option makes sense for you depends on many factors. People with severe physical sensations and those with panic disorder, GAD, and PTSD often have great difficulty at first and may need other medications to see them through the initial detoxification period. When you are further along in the process of tapering and have developed some confidence about your ability to maintain your sense of calm even in anxiety-provoking situations, you may wish to stop the use of all medications.

If you suffer from PTSD or OCD, two anxiety disorders whose symptoms can be improved but rarely entirely ameliorated by any treatment, you may find the use of other medications useful indefinitely, perhaps for many years. You may also want to stay on other medications indefinitely if you have a genetic or biological component to your anxiety. As we previously discussed, there is no specific test that proves the presence of a biological abnormality that causes anxiety. A lifetime of anxiety, or the presence of other family members who have anxiety disorders, strongly suggests that your symptoms are due in part to a biological predisposition to anxiety and that you may benefit from other medications.

3. TAPERING YOUR DOSAGE

Several issues need to be addressed so that you can taper your dosage successfully.

First, it may take a month or two to develop some skill in the use of relaxation techniques and adjust any other medications so that they are as effective as possible. It is reasonable to continue to take your usual dose during this time to allow yourself to prepare to deal with the withdrawal symptoms that will arise when you begin the tapering process.

Second, you must work with your psychiatrist to draw up a schedule of tapering dosages so that you know ahead of time when each reduction will occur. If you have been taking your pills for years, then there is no rush to get off them rapidly. I have found that people are much more successful if they proceed slowly and steadily. If they try to go too rapidly, they become overwhelmed with the intensification of their symptoms and need to return to their original dose just to regain their equilibrium. This can set the entire process back for many months.

Third, each reduction in dose should be quite small in order to minimize the severity of the symptoms of withdrawal and anxiety. I generally reduce the dose by the smallest tablet size available. For example, Xanax comes in 0.25, 0.5, 0.75, and 1.0 milligram tablets. If a person is taking 1.0 milligram of Xanax three times a day, or 3.0 milligrams total at the start of tapering, the first dosage reduction would be down to 1.0 two times a day and 0.75 once a day, or 2.75 milligrams total. It doesn't matter which of the day's doses gets reduced because they are all going to drop to zero at the end. I let patients pick the dose they will reduce based on which will be easier for them. Most find that their anxiety is least in the middle of the day and they decide to reduce those doses first.

Fourth, if you vary your dose each day depending on your level of anxiety, you should start the initial dosage size at a level at which you will be fully comfortable. There is no point in making the first month any harder than it needs to be.

Fifth, you should reduce your dose only once a month. Most

people find that they experience no change the first day or two after a reduction. By the second or third day, however, they have begun to have an intensification of their symptoms of anxiety due to physical withdrawal from the drug. This intensification usually lasts about two weeks or so. Then the withdrawal symptoms ease up and the symptoms of anxiety return to their previous level. Many people use the last two weeks of the month to gather their emotional strength to prepare themselves for the next reduction in dosage.

Sixth, you should stick to your schedule no matter what happens in your life. Though many people want to skip a planned reduction if situations arise that lead them to be more anxious, the hard fact is that life is always presenting anxiety-provoking situations. When difficult circumstances arise, it is important to put the other skills that you have been practicing to good use.

I make an exception to this rule when there has been a sudden death of someone close to a patient, in part because I think patients are justifiably preoccupied with their thoughts and feelings about the person who died and it seems inappropriate to insist on keeping the focus on the tapering process. Also, the death of someone close is a time-limited event. A brief delay in the tapering process is only a brief hiatus. It doesn't necessarily mean that a person is having problems managing anxiety. In fact, many people find that their interest in getting off benzodiazepines actually increases after someone close to them dies because they realize that life is short and they want to live it as best they can.

Seventh, it's important not to take a dose smaller than the agreed-upon dose on "easy days," even though it may seem as if you are doing better than expected. When you do so, it becomes all too easy to make up for these "easy days" by taking extras on "hard days." Making alterations in the tapering schedule because of external events perpetuates the cycle of focusing on anxiety and modulating it with more or less medication. This in turn leads right back into using anxiety as a compass in life, which is exactly what you are trying to get away from.

Some patients do not want to taper their dosage slowly, saying they want to get the whole thing over with as soon as possible. Although it is possible to withdraw from benzodiazepines without any major physical effects much more rapidly than by making the small monthly reduction suggested, people must also learn to develop other methods of managing their anxiety so that they will not be overwhelmed when they finally stop their pills.

I recommend a rapid taper for people who are taking a much higher dose than I prescribe, either by prematurely using up what the pharmacy gives them or by obtaining it from friends or on the street, and for people who are also hooked on other drugs as well. For these people, a slow taper cannot be accomplished because we can't work reliably and honestly together while they are abusing the drug. A rapid taper, though exceedingly unpleasant, is the only possible option. Sometimes inpatient hospitalization proves necessary for this. Even a rapid taper should be gradual enough to avoid seizures.

4. DEVELOPING ALTERNATIVE METHODS TO MANAGE ANXIETY

Though they may be unpleasant and difficult to carry out, the first three steps are relatively straightforward. Developing alternative methods to manage anxiety, however, is a much more complex task. As we discussed, one of the problems with the regular use of benzodiazepines is that other methods of coping with anxiety are rarely used. Confronting anxiety without the aid of benzodiazepines will require you to behave in new ways. Although these new behaviors may seem awkward and even uncomfortable at first, they offer you the potential to begin to regain control of your life. What are some other successful ways of managing anxiety?

Table 3, derived from the work of George Clum, author of *Coping with Panic,* lists many alternative anxiety reduction strategies.[1] As can be seen, they vary tremendously. Some are primarily mental, some are physical. Some can be carried out quite simply, some are more complex. Some take a few seconds or minutes, others may take hours. Some, like splashing water on your face or practicing a relaxation technique, only change your physical and mental state. Others, such as reading, working on a hobby, or talking with others, can also provide some emotional and intellectual satisfaction in addition to their effect on anxiety.

In order to manage your anxiety differently, then, you need to select some specific methods that seem sensible and feasible to you and then practice them. You can choose some of the methods that

TABLE 3

ANXIETY COPING STRATEGIES*

Relaxation techniques	Listening to music
Consulting a professional	Working on a crossword puzzle
Medication	Working around the house
Exercising	Playing a game
Telling yourself it will pass	Watching television
Distracting yourself mentally	Reading a book
Working	Talking to other people
Splashing water on your face	Letting the symptoms happen
Changing positions	Eating or drinking
Going outside for fresh air	Leaving the situation
Engaging in sexual activity	Having someone accompany you
Working on a hobby	Avoiding the situation

*Adapted from Clum 1990

are listed in Table 3. You can also ask other people what they do to manage anxiety. Perhaps you can brainstorm some new ones for yourself. Try to choose at least two that not only offer some relaxation during the activity but also interest you apart from any anxiety-reduction qualities. As we saw in the cases of Janet and Marilyn, these activities can be a bridge between your focus early in treatment on reducing anxiety and your focus later in treatment on developing activities that are meaningful and satisfying to you in your life.

You may need to try a number of different methods before finding those that work for you. Remember that you want to use only those methods that will work in the short and long run, and those that increase your self-esteem and self-efficacy. Assess your inner state whenever you have performed one of your new methods. Do you feel less anxious? Do you feel that you are in charge?

5. CONFRONTING THE SOURCES OF YOUR ANXIETY

The previous four steps, though they may have been difficult, have been only preliminary steps to the main task: facing the sources of your anxiety and working on real solutions to them. This will obviously be a difficult challenge—which is probably one reason you have been avoiding it for as long as you've been taking your pills. Now, however, you have mastered four tasks that probably once felt impossible: You've made a firm commitment to stop your usage, you've practiced relaxation techniques so that you know you can tolerate some sensations of anxiety without being overwhelmed, you've reduced your usage, and you've developed some other methods of managing your anxiety. There is no reason you can't be successful at this stage as well.

As we have discussed, there are two main sources of a person's anxiety: current stresses and traumatic experiences from the past. Current stresses often include such things as conflicts in relationships, difficulties at work, medical problems, or entering a new period in one's life that may require new skills and a different way of doing things. Traumatic experiences that occurred in the past that still lead to anxiety may include sexual, physical, and emotional abuse, and neglect of emotional needs due to parental divorce, alcohol use, premature death, sickness, and poverty.

Most people initially address current stresses—for several reasons. First, current stresses usually cause some obvious distress and limitations and they call for solutions right away. Second, most people do not want to dredge up old memories and feelings about painful times from the past because they can see no useful purpose to it. Third, many people do not recognize that past events may still be influencing them today.

All of these reasons are sensible, and I generally recommend that people address the current issues that are troubling to them when we reach this stage of their treatment. I also know that it is generally pointless to discuss old experiences unless a person can connect them to real events in their current life. These connections are most usefully made in the later stages of therapy.

As we have seen, sometimes the source of anxiety is not clear, causing some people to jump to the conclusion that there is no cause for their symptoms and that they have a "chemical imbalance." Although it is difficult and can seem pointless, it is essential to stretch one's mind and consider any possible source of anxiety. This is best accomplished with an unstructured approach in which a person says whatever comes to mind and then follows up the thoughts that emerge with the aid of the psychotherapist.

6. MAKING PROGRESS

People make progress and can begin to feel better with each step in the process. If you persevere, you are sure to make some headway in solving the problems that lead you to be anxious. Progress won't necessarily come easily or right away. If you're like the rest of the human race, you'll make mistakes and have setbacks. Maybe you'll figure out some way to communicate with your spouse about an issue that you've never been able to discuss together, only to have other issues arise. Maybe you'll shift something in your life in response to a medical problem, only to have another problem crop up. Or perhaps you'll change jobs only to find your new job causes you more stress than the old. Once you begin to make some changes, however, you will begin to see that other changes are possible. Once you have broken the paralysis caused by benzodiazepines, you will realize that many things that you never considered for yourself are possible.

Don't give up too early! The biggest problem you may have once you have begun to make some changes is that you may decide to be satisfied with less than you are capable of creating for yourself. Many people who get off benzodiazepines and learn new ways of managing their anxiety stop their treatment prematurely, making only minimal attempts to learn about and put into perspective unresolved feelings from previous traumatic experiences. While it is true that work on old feelings is difficult, stopping treatment at this time is like spending all day preparing dinner and only eating the soup. While your acute hunger pains may be relieved, you'll feel truly satisfied only when you stay for the full course.

Many people have spent ten, twenty, or even fifty years fighting the symptoms of anxiety and repressing the memories of the traumatic situations that cause them. People who have managed anxiety in one way for decades do not easily shift to new ways in a few weeks of good intentions. Many need one, two, or even more years of therapy to feel that they have sufficiently understood old issues and resolved leftover feelings so that they feel confident in their decision to stop.

There are no "criteria" to help decide when a person should stop seeing a therapist. Most people balance the time, effort, and money involved in therapy with an assessment of how they are

232 Overcoming Anxiety *without* Tranquilizers

feeling and functioning and the possible gains from further treatment, but the decision is essentially one of personal preference.

7. TAKING CHARGE

Freedom from benzodiazepines, freedom from the narrow, constricted life that they promote, freedom from worrying about anxiety all the time—all these occur in people who embark on the recovery process from dependency.

Life itself will not allow you to be free from anxiety. After all, normal anxiety is an essential human experience that alerts us to challenges in our life that we need to prepare for and respond to. But once you are free from benzodiazepines, you no longer need to use anxiety as a compass; now you can use it more efficiently, as an early warning system. You can be the director in charge of your life, deciding how to respond in ways that will be best for you in the short and long run, rather than being stuck with just finding ways to make your anxiety less.

· 12 ·

ALCOHOL AND BENZOS

The use of benzodiazepines and alcohol frequently become entwined in the lives of people with anxiety disorders.[1] Part of the reason for this is that this class of drugs may have a positive mood effect in people who have become dependent on alcohol.[2] In this chapter I will outline four common patterns. They are quite different, and each requires a different emphasis in treatment. If you use benzodiazepines now, and are now or have ever used alcohol excessively, you and your psychiatrist may need to incorporate some treatment of your drinking into your treatment plan.

Although the body can generally tolerate excessive ingestion of either alcohol or benzodiazepines, profound respiratory depression and even death can result from simultaneous ingestion of even small doses of both. The combination of the two not infrequently results in a completed suicide.[3]

WHEN ANXIETY LEADS TO ALCOHOL DEPENDENCY AND BENZO USE

Some people experience chronic anxiety from an early age, due to biological factors, overwhelming traumatic experiences, or both. One of the more maladaptive ways people manage this form of chronic anxiety is to "medicate" it with alcohol. Though they may drink what appears to be only a small amount, their functioning can still be impaired in either subtle or obvious ways. For example, they may confine their drinking to periods when they are not working, perhaps justifying their alcohol use by saying that they only drink "responsibly" or "socially." On closer examination, however, it is clear that they are using the alcohol to minimize their anxiety when they don't have the structure of a job to contain their anxiety and take their minds off it. And, of course, some people with anxiety disorders drink large amounts of alcohol daily and have the kinds of problems that are associated with alcoholism, such as depression, health problems, impaired job performance, and disrupted relationships.

Whether the amount of alcohol is large or small, it is very difficult for the sufferers of chronic anxiety to stop drinking unless they also get some help with their anxiety. These people have a double problem: in addition to the addictive qualities of alcohol itself, they have a specific disorder that is contributing to their alcohol use. They are at great risk for developing dependence on benzodiazepines when they attempt to stop drinking alcohol.

Three factors contribute to this risk. In the first place, people who manage anxiety with alcohol have chronic anxiety, which we know is exactly the problem that most frequently leads to chronic use. Second, these people have clearly opted to ingest a substance as a means of managing anxiety. This is different from adopting other maladaptive strategies, such as restricting their lives or depending on other people—to say nothing of the constructive ways of managing anxiety, such as relaxation techniques, therapy, and working directly on the sources of anxiety. The pattern of trying to "fix" uncomfortable feelings by ingesting something can be a hard one to change. Third, "rebound" anxiety is one of the effects of withdrawal from alcohol. Since they drink to minimize anxiety in the first place, it becomes doubly hard for these people to stop drinking without using something else to help them with their symptoms of anxiety. For these reasons, people who use alcohol to medicate their anxiety have an even harder time stopping drinking than people who have not experienced chronic anxiety. And they are far more likely to use benzodiazepines when they do try to stop drinking.

It can be difficult to distinguish alcohol use that is driven by anxiety from alcoholism plain and simple. One helpful clue is whether other family members experience anxiety. If they do, it may be that the person is drinking in part to medicate anxiety. Another clue that anxiety is the underlying disorder is its presence prior to the alcohol use. Also, an anxiety disorder is likely present if a person has difficulty with anxiety for more than a few weeks after stopping the use of alcohol. Finally, people with long-term difficulty managing their anxiety may wish to continue benzodiazepine use beyond the acute period of alcohol withdrawal.

This was the case with Bob. While he was growing up, he generally felt somewhat anxious, even though he wasn't afraid of anything in particular, such as dying or monsters in the dark. He began biting his nails at the age of six. His parents had to put tape on his thumbs so that he wouldn't suck them at night. In fourth and fifth grade he often had a "nervous stomach" before going to school, even though he usually did well once there. His parents drank alcohol regularly on nights and weekends but never had any obvious problems, such as car accidents while drinking or fights at home. When he was sixteen, Bob often had a beer or two when he finished his part-time work as a dishwasher. He also began smoking marijuana on weekends around this time. He felt more relaxed and better able to have a good time when he was drinking or smoking marijuana.

By age nineteen Bob had begun to develop an ulcer, and he frequently took antacids to treat it. His alcohol use increased greatly at this time; he began drinking nightly and having a six-pack or two on weekends. He did well in school, however, because he studied hard at night and on weekends before he started drinking. After college, Bob got a job selling encyclopedias and did quite well because of his strong ambition and motivation. However, when he wasn't working, he generally spent his time drinking or using marijuana. When he got together with friends, he invariably drank. Once in a while Bob stopped drinking for a day or a week, and once even for a month. However, he would soon start feeling anxious, restless, or dissatisfied and resume the use of alcohol.

During a routine physical exam when Bob was twenty-five, his physician noticed that his liver was tender. Bob was relieved when his blood tests came back normal, but he was still surprised that his alcohol use was causing some physical effects. He was somewhat shaken up and decided to stop drinking. Over the next several weeks, however, he was aware of feeling anxious. He went back to see his physician, who prescribed a low dose of Klonopin. The medication was very helpful in minimizing his anxiety, and Bob was able to avoid using alcohol. One night he went with his friends to a nightclub, however, and had a couple of beers. He felt guilty the next day for drinking, and also for drinking while taking the Klonopin, which his doctor had warned him against. Over the next month he went out drinking two more times but skipped his doses of Klonopin to avoid combining them.

When his physician learned that Bob was drinking again, he stopped prescribing Klonopin. He explained that the simultaneous use of the two can cause severe respiratory depression to the point of death. Bob told the doctor that he probably would drink more if he didn't have the Klonopin, but the doctor still refused to prescribe more. Bob then began to drink again, and his use gradually escalated to its previous level.

At the insistence of his girlfriend, who wanted him to stop drinking or at least to drink less, Bob consulted a psychiatrist. The psychiatrist started him on Ativan, stating that this would help his anxiety and would consequently help him to stop drinking. For the first month Bob didn't drink at all. Over the next several months, however, he did begin to drink again, although he drank less than before using Ativan. The psychiatrist continually urged him to stop drinking and attend AA, but Bob never seemed to follow through.

Both doctors tried to help Bob but neither was successful. His family doctor identified a problem with drinking that needed to be addressed but didn't see that Bob also had long-term problems with anxiety and that the anxiety needed to be a focus of treatment. When Bob began using alcohol, and the Klonopin at the same time, his doctor lumped all the problems under the heading of "drug abuse," refused to participate in maintaining the abuse, and essentially threw Bob out of the office. Because the doctor missed the central role played by Bob's anxiety and thus did not steer him to appropriate drug-free treatment, Bob stood little chance of successfully staying off alcohol.

Bob's psychiatrist, on the other hand, saw that Bob needed ongoing help with anxiety but didn't help him to see that ingesting substances was not a good long-term solution. By continuing to write prescriptions in spite of his continued drinking, the psychiatrist enabled Bob to avoid dealing with anxiety. Many people with long-standing difficulties managing anxiety seek prescriptions for benzodiazepines when stopping their use of alcohol. They become a substitute for the alcohol.

Bob needed help with all three problems: alcoholism, anxiety, and benzodiazepine dependency. He needed to address his alcohol dependence directly through regular attendance at Alcoholics Anonymous meetings. He needed to learn how to manage his anxiety more effectively and taper his drug use. Once all three problems became a focus of treatment he was able to stay substance-free and overcome being controlled by anxiety.

If you struggle with anxiety and alcohol abuse, don't fall into the trap of substituting one poison for another. Aim your treatment at the real problem—anxiety—and leave addictive substances behind.

WHEN ANXIETY LEADS TO BENZO DEPENDENCE AND ALCOHOL USE

Some people with anxiety use benzodiazepines for a period of time and then begin to use alcohol intermittently. They sometimes skip their pill when they know they are going to drink, in an effort to be safe or "responsible." Nevertheless, the easy substitution clarifies the role that both play: to medicate the symptoms of anxiety. People would recognize the negative aspects of regular benzodiazepine use more easily if they thought about how the substitution would work in reverse—namely, having an alcoholic beverage three times a day to combat anxiety, and an extra drink on "really difficult days."

Carol primarily used benzodiazepines to treat anxiety but then started using alcohol as well. Anxiety affected many members of her family, including her mother, an aunt, and two brothers. She had an uncle who was an alcoholic, and one of her brothers had abused alcohol for years before finally stopping drinking. Carol had never been aware of being anxious, although she recognized that she was somewhat shy and introverted. When she broke up with her boyfriend of six years, she had difficulty coping. She had moved out of her family's home to live with him and had never been on her own before. Because of her anxiety she was prescribed Valium by her family doctor. Carol used it only once or twice a day, but she didn't seem to be able to get along without it. Although she had used alcohol only sparingly in the past, she now fell into the habit of having a few drinks whenever she went out with friends. Then she had a minor traffic accident when she had been drinking. The court ordered a substance abuse evaluation. A psychologist evaluated Carol's alcohol use but also questioned her closely about her anxiety, her use of Valium, and her feelings about the breakup of her relationship. He concluded not only that Carol's use of alcohol was inappropriate but also that she needed to work in psychotherapy on her feelings about the breakup, on her anxiety, and on more constructive ways of managing her anxiety.

Unlike Bob, who used alcohol to manage his anxiety and then added benzodiazepines to the mix, Carol was among the people who use these drugs for a period of time and then begin to use alcohol intermittently. She needed to be helped primarily by focusing in psychotherapy on her anxiety and use of benzodiazepines. Once she realized that her alcohol use was being driven by her anxiety and that it was inappropriate, she stopped drinking without any specific treatment.

If you are like Carol, and occasionally use alcohol while still taking pills, you are playing with fire. Besides the risk of dangerous respiratory depression, your alcohol use is a sign that your current approach to your problem with anxiety—i.e., benzodiazepines—is ineffective. You need a new approach to help you with anxiety. Consider getting a consultation or a second opinion with a psychiatrist to draw up a new plan.

WHEN DEPENDENCE ON ALCOHOL PRECEDES BENZO USE

Anxiety is not the only reason that people use alcohol in self-destructive ways. However, if people use alcohol regularly enough to become physically dependent on it, they will experience anxiety as a withdrawal symptom if they stop drinking for any reason. If these people are prescribed benzodiazepines to minimize the anxiety, they may begin to believe that the drugs "help" them stop drinking. If the drugs in turn are stopped, however, these people experience rebound anxiety again and are very likely to drink again. The prescription of benzodiazepines for an alcohol user merely substitutes dependence on one drug for another.

Fred often said that he was born with a bottle in each hand. He had first tried alcohol at age eleven, began occasional use at fifteen, and by seventeen was regularly drinking a six-pack a day. When he reached his early twenties he began drinking hard liquor and on occasion consumed as much as a pint in one day. He lost several jobs because of arguments with bosses and co-workers that were directly or indirectly related to his alcohol use. His family and friends were not surprised when he had a car accident while drinking. Because of his physical injuries, Fred had to stay in the hospital for several days.

Deprived of alcohol, he experienced sweating, shakes, insomnia, and anxiety. His doctor prescribed Librium, which relieved a number of his unpleasant symptoms. The doctor referred him to a psychiatrist after he was discharged and also gave him a prescription for Librium. Fred was still experiencing anxiety when he saw the psychiatrist five days later. The psychiatrist recommended that Fred attend AA but also told him to stay on the Librium to help with his "generalized anxiety disorder" so that he wouldn't drink again. Fred attended AA sporadically over the next several months, but he continued to drink alcohol intermittently as well. His psychiatrist continued the prescription of the Librium in the hope that this would decrease Fred's alcohol use.

Anxiety usually occurs when people who are dependent on alcohol stop drinking. This anxiety should not be treated as a psychiatric illness, or given a psychiatric diagnosis. The prescription of benzodiazepines prevents the person from facing and working on their real problems—namely, the abuse of alcohol. The psychiatrist should have focused on helping Fred achieve and maintain abstinence by chipping away at his resistance to attend AA meetings more regularly, pointing out the consequences of his alcohol use on his health and his difficulty keeping a job, and refusing to prescribe Librium.

If you are actively struggling with maintaining sobriety from alcohol, benzodiazepines will not provide any real aid. Commit yourself more strongly to effective treatment to help you to stop drinking.

WHEN ALCOHOL AND BENZOS ARE USED AS DRUGS OF ABUSE

Benzodiazepines can produce euphoric feelings and a "high" in some people, and so they use them specifically for that purpose. As noted previously, they can also be used simultaneously with other drugs as part of a regular pattern of drug abuse.

Alice, for instance, began using drugs at the age of fourteen when she started using diet pills. Although she used them to keep thin, she also liked the extra "boost" of energy that they gave her. Sometimes it was hard for her to fall asleep at night, however, and she would occasionally sneak some of her parents' wine. By age sixteen she was drinking alcohol regularly and using marijuana, and at nineteen she began using cocaine. Over the next three years Alice used as much cocaine as she could pay for. If she couldn't get cocaine she would sometimes use speed. She bought Valium and Ativan on the street and took them to help her "come down" from the highs produced by the other drugs. She still used alcohol regularly, both to get high and to slow her down from the speed and cocaine.

Alice went through two hospitalizations, when she was twenty-two and twenty-four, for drug abuse. Each time she was given Xanax to help treat her "anxiety." Both times Alice started using drugs again almost as soon as she was discharged. At twenty-five her intravenous cocaine use resulted in such a severe case of hepatitis that she required hospitalization for several weeks. Alice vowed never to use drugs again. Upon discharge, she lived for eight months in a treatment house with six other adults who were trying to stop drug use; the house was staffed with clinicians who specialized in providing treatment of people with severe substance abuse disorders. When Alice finally moved out, she was able to maintain her sobriety by attending AA and Narcotics Anonymous (NA) groups daily. Eventually, she was able to find and maintain employment working in a retail clothing store.

Alice used benzodiazepines as merely one of a mixture of drugs. The number of people who abuse this class of drugs in this way is, thankfully, quite small. Their treatment is difficult, but straightforward: to create as much support as possible to achieve and maintain abstinence from drug use.

If you are using benzodiazepines and other drugs to alter your thoughts and feelings, you may think that they somehow improve your life. Positive alternatives to drug use exist, however, if you seek them out.

CONCLUSION

Many people who use both benzodiazepines and alcohol do not fit neatly into one of these four patterns, of course, such as a person with long-standing anxiety who also uses them as drugs of abuse. In general, the evaluation of someone who uses both needs to separate out three components: whether there is a primary anxiety disorder present; whether alcohol and benzodiazepines are used as drugs of abuse; and whether alcohol is being used to "treat" the anxiety.

It is essential to perform a complete evaluation of a person's anxiety and their substance use in order to develop a sensible plan that addresses both problems. Besides the evaluation for anxiety described in chapter 8, an evaluation of a person's substance use includes learning the amount of any current use; when alcohol was first used; the pattern and amount of use over the years (e.g., daily or binge drinking; two beers or a fifth of vodka); the degree of preoccupation with alcohol; any attempts to control the amount or frequency of drinking and whether there have been periods of sobriety; whether it has caused any disruptions in relationships or employment; whether it has caused medical problems such as blackouts, hangovers, ulcers, hepatitis, seizures, or delirium tremens; whether it has caused an involvement with the legal system such as arrests for driving under the influence of alcohol; the abuse of other substances such as marijuana, cocaine, or narcotics; previous treatment; family history of alcohol use; the patient's insight into alcohol as a problem and his willingness to engage in treatment.

A comprehensive treatment plan to address each of these areas is necessary in order to achieve success. It is essential to utilize all necessary treatment modalities in order to achieve and maintain abstinence from alcohol, and in all cases, benzodiazepines need to be tapered and stopped. Additionally, treatment directed at the anxiety disorder must also occur.

· 13 ·

THE LAST WORD ON BENZOS

I find it sad and frustrating to see people waste years of their life under the influence of benzodiazepines: young people who limit their choices prematurely; middle-aged people who slide into a restricted life; and the older person who settles for much less than is possible. These feelings motivated me to understand what causes the Benzo Blues and how to lift oneself out of them. I hope that you now understand why you should not rely on benzodiazepines for the relief of chronic anxiety. They are ineffective; they cause physical and psychological dependency as well as other direct and indirect side effects; they blunt your body's signal of anxiety about issues that need to be addressed and resolved, thereby sabotaging your motivation to seek treatment that may be more difficult but is far more effective. Most important, they deprive you of the chance to benefit from engaging in new challenges and opportunities because you are instead preoccupied with avoiding anxiety and are mired in the Benzo Blues.

I also hope you see that there is a way out. Like many others who have become dependent on benzodiazepines, you can have a life that is satisfying and meaningful. You can have a life in which you are in control.

Although my reasoning may be sound, you may still be reluctant to taper your usage and learn new ways to manage and overcome anxiety. The decision to change from benzodiazepines to the use of other ways to manage anxiety can be scary for many reasons. You may feel it is better to keep walking down the same old path—though it is unsatisfying and discouraging, it is predictable. The path of change may have more hope, but you will have to face uncomfortable problems and much that is unknown. Perhaps your anxiety will get worse. Perhaps you will need to start taking benzodiazepines again, this time with a feeling of failure to accompany the anxiety. Perhaps you are afraid to jeopardize whatever possible aspects of your life that you have achieved.

To help you overcome your reluctance to choose the path of hope and change, I offer a piece of advice that will help you take the first step and make the commitment to get off your pills: Take a written inventory of your relationships, activities, and feelings that make up your life now, and make a second list of what you would like them to be in the future.

Try to use the feelings of dissatisfaction that you feel as you compare the two not to fuel the paralysis that benzodiazepines promote but as a stimulus to try to make things better for yourself. Don't let these drugs keep you on the path of discouragement and hopelessness. Although you will almost assuredly encounter difficulties on the path of change, you will meet them as your own master, not as the victim of anxiety and medication.

I hope you choose the path of change and make the commitment to get off benzodiazepines. If you feel unable to do so at this time, however, pick a date in the not-too-distant future when you will raise this issue with yourself again. Don't wait too long—your life is waiting.

AFTERWORD: FINDING A PSYCHIATRIST

$\underset{\text{It}}{\LARGE I}$ can be difficult to find the right psychiatrist. None of us is entirely comfortable in baring our soul—especially when we are having problems. Nevertheless, you are going to need to work with one to get off benzodiazepines and start taking charge of your life.

If you are prescribed the drugs from your primary care provider, you might consider sharing your concern about your dependency and ask for a referral to a psychiatrist who can help you to get off them. If you don't feel comfortable asking for a referral, in most cities there are medical schools and hospitals that can give you names. Rural communities have fewer psychiatrists, but their names can also be obtained from a nearby hospital or mental health center. Your third-party payer, such as an insurance company or HMO, may require you to see a psychiatrist who is on their panel.

The real problem isn't finding a psychiatrist—it's finding one who feels right to you. Working with a psychiatrist is extremely personal, and it's important that your choice be a good one for you. There are three aspects you should consider in your search.

First, you should feel confident about the psychiatrist's professional qualifications. All psychiatrists have gone to medical school, and the vast majority have finished three or more years of specialty training after that as well. While most are quite proficient in prescribing medications, however, they may have very different views on how medication might be of help to you. Make sure they don't see medications as the only form of treatment that can be helpful for you.

Second, there are many personal qualities in a psychiatrist that you need to take into account. You should feel comfortable with the age, race, and gender of anyone you see. You should also feel comfortable with them as a person. Some people like a psychiatrist who appears confident, while others may find the same one arrogant. A psychiatrist can appear reserved and thoughtful to one patient, while another patient may feel only coldness and distance. Some people want a psychiatrist with a good sense of humor, while others might find this unprofessional. The work together will go best if you and your psychiatrist make a good "fit," and you are the only one who can decide if the fit is right for you.

Finally, explain that you want to come off benzodiazepines, but that you want to do it slowly, sensibly, and carefully. If she suggests adding another medication, ask specifically how it is supposed to help you, how long you will take it, and what the side effects are. Explain that you want to live a life in which you are in control, not your anxiety. Ask if she is familiar with behavioral techniques that can help you learn to manage the symptoms of anxiety without using benzodiazepines. Most important, ask if she will help you to learn about and resolve the issues that are leading to your anxiety. Many psychiatrists are not adequately trained in working with people in long-term psychotherapy to identify the experiences that led to anxiety and resolve the feelings that remain from those experiences. And, unfortunately, many third-party payers are refusing to pay psychiatrists to do this work, believing that other professionals can perform it for a lower fee. It is reasonable, though perhaps not ideal, to work with a psychiatrist on tapering the benzodiazepines while at the same time working with a nonphysician psychotherapist on learning how to manage the symptoms of anxiety and identifying and resolving the experiences that lead to your anxiety. If you work with a psychiatrist and a nonphysician therapist, all three of you should agree on the overall goal of treatment and communicate freely among one another throughout its course.

When you first see a psychiatrist, therefore, while she is evaluating you, you should be doing your own evaluation. In truth, you are the employer, and the psychiatrist is interviewing for the job—only if the person feels "right" to you should you sign on for more. This decision can usually be made after one session, but it is reasonable to schedule two or three meetings in an "extended" evaluation to insure that the two of you will work well together. You should agree to start your work together only if you are satisfied with all three areas: the right professional qualifications, the right "fit," and a sensible comprehensive treatment plan. If the fit isn't right—confront it directly. You do yourself no favors to stay with someone about whom you don't feel confident.

APPENDIX: THE RESEARCH ON BENZOS

The research on benzodiazepines is voluminous because of their popularity and the controversy surrounding their use. It is filled with conflicting claims by different investigators, each proclaiming to state the "truth" about benzodiazepines. In this appendix I will review the literature and the conflicting findings. This close examination of the scientific literature will enable us to see the reasons why different investigators disagree and what it teaches us about anxiety and benzodiazepines.

ELEMENTS OF SCIENTIFIC RESEARCH

The disagreements that range between scientists hinge on differing interpretations of the same basic evidence that is published in scientific journals. This is especially true in any study of psychiatric problems (as opposed to more objectively quantifiable phenomena such as survival rates in cancer patients treated with different forms of chemotherapy) because there are so many complex issues to take into account. As a first step, let's look closely at the elements of any study investigating benzodiazepines. This will help us to understand how to interpret the validity of individual studies.

Financial Support for the Study often colors the results before the experiment is even started. Pharmaceutical companies must produce evidence that their drugs are effective before the Federal Drug Administration (FDA) will allow them to sell them on the open market. The scientists who work for the drug companies tend to narrow the focus on the initial studies in order to demonstrate that their drugs are effective for at least one problem. By and large, drug side effects are minimized. In the summary of their work, pharmaceutical company researchers often go on to speculate about other possible uses for the drug that is under investigation. The best and most objective studies are done by researchers who are independently supported by universities or government grants, since they tend to take a much wider and more critical look at the drugs that they study.

Subject Selection is an especially important issue. How are people recruited for the study? Vastly different results can be obtained about the same drug depending on how the subjects are recruited. One common method occurs at university hospitals and clinics, where physicians perform research on the patients who seek them out for treatment. This is very different from recruiting subjects through newspaper ads who are then paid through funds from a drug company. A recruitment advertisement skews the sample toward people who have not benefitted from treatment by their current doctor. In addition, a patient's motivation to comply with the efforts of the investigator can be increased if they are paid. Both of these practices may alter the composition of the group of subjects to the point that they are not representative of a doctor's practice. While the method of subject recruitment matters little if the drug is an antibiotic being tested against infection, it can have a more substantial effect in psychiatric drug treatment evaluations because the phenomena being studied are more subjective and dependent on the patient's report.

A good study describes the *inclusion* criteria, which are the characteristics of the patients that led them to be selected for the study. For example, the inclusion criteria might be "all patients over twenty-one admitted to the emergency room in the first three months of 1995 who were given a diagnosis of any anxiety disorder and who were prescribed benzos by the emergency room physician." Studies should also describe the *exclusion* criteria, which is a list of the conditions that lead to the exclusion of some of the patients chosen for study. Subjects are often excluded if they have epilepsy, a thyroid disorder, other psychiatric disorders such as depression or schizophrenia, are pregnant or suicidal, have a drug or alcohol dependency, or are involved elsewhere in active psychiatric treatment such as psychotherapy.

Psychiatric researchers have also realized in the last twenty years that the psychiatric diagnoses of the patients in the study must be accurate and uniform, because any variability in the subjects' psychiatric conditions makes it virtually impossible to generalize the results to other patients and studies. Much of the psychiatric literature examining anxiety prior to 1970 is virtually worthless because diagnoses of anxiety were made so haphazardly and included people who had schizophrenia, depression, and alcohol dependence. Many studies that examined the usefulness of benzodiazepines for anxiety made no attempt to define the specific characteristics of their subjects' anxiety disorders. This neglect led to studies in which patients with panic disorder were lumped with those who had generalized anxiety disorder and even obsessive-compulsive disorder.

Researchers should describe the personal characteristics of the subject in order for doctors to determine whether or not the results of the study are likely to apply to one of their patients. Important descriptive details include age, sex, race, marital status, economic status, the coexistence of any medical problems, duration of symptoms, and history of previous treatments. It is also important to eliminate people with medical disorders such as a thyroid or liver disease that might confound the effects of a drug. Good studies document the psychiatric and medical conditions that lead to the exclusion of people from the study.

Assessment. It is obviously essential to define how the subjects' symptoms of anxiety change as a result of the drug treatment. This is generally accomplished through the use of a rating scale, which is usually a list of symptoms filled out by the patient or researcher before, during, and after the study. It is important that the rating scale have *reliability* and *validity*. The reliability of a rating scale refers to the degree to which different raters can use the same scale and obtain the same results. Validity means that the results obtained in the study accurately reflect the condition of the person being studied. The simultaneous use of rating scales by both the doctor/researcher and the patient/subject has demonstrated that there is sometimes a significant difference between the two. The best results use multiple rating scales in order to define the change in the patients' condition as completely as possible. It is also important to assess the condition of any patient who leaves the study prematurely.

Study Design. There are many variations in the structure of any study that enhance or detract from the validity of its findings. No study can evaluate the effectiveness of a medication without a *control* group. This is a second group of people who are matched by age, sex, race, weight, diagnosis, severity of anxiety, and other factors and who receive a different treatment, such as another drug, a certain form of psychotherapy, or a placebo (a pill that looks like the drug but contains no active ingredients in it). A control group is necessary because simply participating in a study and taking medication can have many effects, regardless of the drug or treatment that is being studied.

Studies should be *double-blind,* which means that neither the subjects nor the evaluators of the subjects' condition know which patients are receiving which treatment until the code is broken at the completion of the study. This is best accomplished when independent clinicians evaluate the conditions of the subjects and report the results to the principal investigators who are conducting the study. The purpose of using a double-blind design is to minimize any bias by patients or investigators that could influence their assessment of a person's condition. For example, if patients knew that they were taking the active drug, they might be more likely to emphasize an improvement in their symptoms. Similarly, if they knew that they were taking a sugar pill, they might be more likely to report little benefit.

It is important to have an *adequate sample size* of patients. The exact number needed depends on the effects being studied and the complexity of the statistical methods used to analyze the data. Too few may allow the data concerning any supposed effects of the drug found in the study to be skewed as a result of one or two people with an atypical response. Too many can lead to a finding that there is a *statistically* significant difference between the drug being studied and the control treatment, when the amount of difference to any person is so small that it is *clinically* insignificant. Good studies contain a *washout period* during which the subjects stop all their medications before the study has begun in order to insure that any effects seen in the study reflect only the drug that is used. The washout period must be long enough so that the drug itself is out of a person's system and that there are no withdrawal effects remaining. A researcher evaluating medications should attempt to keep their study subjects *off all other medications* so that any effects seen will be due to the drug being studied. Other treatments such as psychotherapy should be limited during the study for the same reason. An *adequate, but not excessive, dosage* of medication is needed to insure that the effects will mimic those experienced by patients in the community. There should be some method to insure that the patient is taking the correct amount of the drug, no more and no less. This may include taking blood levels of the patients at regular intervals throughout the study. The *duration* that the subjects are studied should be appropriate to the treatment given for a particular disorder. Finally, the study needs to document the people who *drop out* of the study and why. If many people drop out of the study because of side effects, reporting only the results of the people who complete the study period can be misleading because the data from people with the positive results will have stayed in while data from those experiencing negative results will have been left out.

Data Analysis. The analysis of the results of a study generally require the use of fairly complex statistics in order to organize the data in a meaningful way. Studies should use statistical methods that are appropriate for the data being analyzed. A full discussion of the importance of statistics and the ways that they can be inappropriately manipulated to fit the researcher's theories is beyond the scope of this book, but it is an important issue nevertheless.

Interpretation of the Results. Researchers should explain and interpret all their results, not just the portion that supports their theories. Additionally, they should not extrapolate their findings beyond what the data show without clearly identifying that they are engaging in speculation. When we examine the study funded by Upjohn to promote Xanax we'll see how researchers can highlight certain portions of their findings and skew their interpretation to get the desired result.

Recommendations to the Reader. Researchers should not make recommendations to the reader beyond what the data supports.

EARLY RESEARCH

There were many articles in the early sixties that supposedly demonstrated that benzodiazepines reduce anxiety.[1] Let's look in detail at one of the studies done in the early years of benzo research to see if the authors' claim that benzos are effective was warranted.

A study published in 1967 and performed by Karl Rickels, a professor of psychiatry at the University of Pennsylvania, and Dean Clyde, of the University of Miami, examined the usefulness of chlordiazepoxide in the treatment of symptoms of anxiety.[2] Forty-two people took chlordiazepoxide and forty-eight took a placebo. Dosages of up to 80 milligrams a day of chlordiazepoxide were given for four weeks. The symptoms of anxiety were measured on the Clyde Mood Scale, which groups the patients' report of their feelings into categories such as friendly, aggressive, clear thinking, sleepy, unhappy, or dizzy. The patients reported their feelings both before and after they received chlordiazepoxide, and the results were compared. Rickels and Clyde reported that the results demonstrated that chlordiazepoxide was better than placebo in improving the symptoms of "anxious" outpatients.

In evaluating this study it is important to note its strengths. The study was double-blind and placebo controlled. Ninety patients is a sufficient number to minimize the likelihood that data from two or three patients with extreme reactions would skew the outcome one way or the other. The study used a specific rating scale to measure improvement.

On the other hand, there were some significant weaknesses in the study as well. The patients were described only as "primarily anxious, frequently somatizing, and often mildly depressed." There were no specific diagnostic, inclusion, or exclusion criteria to insure a homogeneous population. The problem with a study involving so mixed a population is that it is not possible to determine whether the patients who improved actually had a diagnosis of an anxiety disorder. It is possible that chlordiazepoxide only works for those patients who have anxiety with depression or, perhaps, for those with anxiety without depression.

The study noted no criteria that demonstrated that the chlordiazepoxide group was appropriately matched to the placebo group. There was no evidence that the two groups were matched for age, sex, race, marital status, educational level, socioeconomic status, body weight, duration of symptoms, previous response to drugs, presence of a positive life event during the study, or even the level of anxiety. It is very likely that the two groups had some asymmetries in their populations, and it is possible that these asymmetries biased the data.

There was no description of whether other medications or forms of therapy were being used simultaneously by the study participants. Use of other agents such as antidepressants can confound the results of a survey on the usefulness of benzos because some of the effects attributed to the benzos may actually be due to those other drugs. Were some of these patients on other drugs? Were some of them in psychotherapy? The findings might be biased if people in one group, but not the other, were receiving other treatments.

The study contains no description of a washout period. It is possible that some patients stopped taking medications that were helpful to them at the beginning of the study. Patients in the placebo group may have been experiencing withdrawal symptoms if they had been taking benzos or antidepressants when they started the study, substantially worsening their experience of anxiety and falsely magnifying the beneficial effects seen in the chlordiazepoxide group.

There was no mention in the study of people who had dropped out. In many studies, there are dropouts in the placebo group because patients don't want to put up with all the inconvenience of being in a study if they don't feel they are getting better, and dropouts in the active drug group because of side effects. It is important to take the dropout rate into account because an unequal number of dropouts in the two groups can skew the final assessment.

Finally, the Clyde Mood Scale measures only the patients' report of their inner state. There is no evaluation by the researchers of the patients' clinical condition.

These problems significantly undercut the believability of the authors' report that chlordiazepoxide helps "anxious outpatients." The real problem, however, is not just with Rickels's study but arises from the fact that almost all of the early work on benzos suffers from similar deficits.

Because of his belief that the conclusion suggesting that benzodiazepines improve the symptoms of anxiety had not been made in a scientifically sound manner, Kenneth Solomon, a psychiatrist working at the Albany Medical College, examined the quality of research papers studying the usefulness of benzodiazepines in the treatment of anxiety and attempted to find only the best and most objective studies available.[3] All seventy-eight double-blind studies that were available in the French and English literature were evaluated.

All the studies were found to have major flaws. Among the flaws were the inclusion of patients who were suffering from disorders other than anxiety, such as schizophrenia; the lack of definition of what *anxiety* was and how it was to be measured objectively; patients' simultaneous use of other drugs that affect anxiety; inadequate control groups; inadequate dosages of the drug being studied; poor reporting of exactly what dosages the patients were receiving; inadequate duration of study; inadequate washout periods; inadequate sample size; and inadequate analysis of the data due to failure to identify people dropping out.

The article even questioned how truly "blind" such studies can be. Three studies were cited that demonstrate that experienced clinicians are able to correctly guess whether a person is taking an active drug or a placebo from sixty-three to one hundred percent of the time. How valid is a study that purports to be double-blind when the investigators *do* know which drug the patients are taking?

Solomon's conclusion was that "because none of the 78 published double-blind studies are fully adequate, and many are so poorly designed and executed as to be virtually meaningless, the efficacy of the entire group of drugs must be questioned. . . . More and better research is necessary to critically state that these drugs definitely are effective."

LATER RESEARCH

Unfortunately, later work also suffers from significant deficiencies. For example, one study, reported in 1980 by Gary Aden, a researcher at the San Diego Neuropsychiatry Medical Clinic looked at the effects of alprazolam and diazepam compared with placebo.[4] Several measures were used to assess the severity of symptoms in 235 patients who participated in a double-blind study lasting four weeks. The study concluded that alprazolam and diazepam were superior to placebo in overall assessments on the Hamilton Anxiety Rating Scale and two other scales that were rated by a study evaluator, but that there was no difference on the two patients' self-rating scales.

This study had some strengths. There were some appropriate inclusion and exclusion criteria. The investigators used several rating scales to provide a fuller picture. They controlled for some variables. The study was double-blind (even if evaluators could guess correctly some of the time, at least they were trying to be even-handed). They had an adequate sample size. They used adequate dosages.

Nevertheless, there were still some major problems.

Diagnosis. 162 patients were given a diagnosis of anxiety neurosis, while 72 had "mixed anxiety depression" (one had obsessive-compulsive disorder). Once again, it is impossible to determine if the benefit to patients is due to one subset of the patients improving. It is even possible that alprazolam and diazepam help people with depression more than those with anxiety. (In fact, some investigators claim later research shows that alprazolam does help people with depression.)

Rating Scales. Although the abstract (a brief summary of findings that appears at the beginning of every scientific research paper) reports that "alprazolam was more effective than placebo and essentially equivalent to diazepam," this is only true of the scales rated by the study evaluators. As noted, the scales of the ratings by patients failed to demonstrate any difference among the three! The authors acknowledge this only with the brief comment that this finding is "frequently seen in studies of this type."

This presents two serious problems. First, it is disingenuous for the researchers to write in the abstract that alprazolam and diazepam were more effective than placebo when some measurements did not demonstrate any great effectiveness. It is even more objectionable when the authors acknowledge that this occurs "frequently." Secondly, doesn't it tell us something when patients don't notice the same degree of improvement as the evaluators do? Shouldn't we all take notice if patients "frequently" rate medications as less effective than the evaluators? Why should we assume that the evaluators' ratings are more accurate than those of patients? Wouldn't it be just as accurate to conclude that "patients found no benefit from the use of either alprazolam or diazepam beyond that achieved by placebo"?

Confounding Variables. There was no mention of whether patients had received psychotherapy in the past or whether they received any during the study.

Duration of Study. The duration of the study was for only twenty-eight days. Yet ninety percent of these patients had symptoms of anxiety for more than one year. Is a medication that supposedly works for a few weeks (at least from the evaluators' point of view) a sensible treatment for a disorder that is clearly a more chronic disorder? This question isn't even addressed.

Washout. This study had a washout period, but it lasted only one week. This is a standard period of time for most studies. We know from Lader's work that withdrawal symptoms from benzodiazepines can, and usually do, last for several weeks. The same is also true for many antidepressants. As a result, therefore, many patients would have started the study in the midst of an intense period of anxiety due primarily to a discontinuance syndrome. Regardless of the effect of an underlying anxiety disorder, relief from the symptoms of withdrawal would be obtained only in the groups that got alprazolam or diazepam not in the group that got placebo. This relief would be noted by the study patients as "improvement," bias the results, and make benzodiazepines appear more effective than they really are.

David Barlow, a psychiatrist who has written extensively about anxiety, reviewed this study and many others performed between 1978 and 1988.[5] He evaluated all double-blind placebo-controlled studies in which the investigators used the same method for measuring how patients' symptoms changed during the investigation, the Hamilton Anxiety Rating Scale. The Hamilton Scale measures the severity of anxiety by means of a checklist of the symptoms of anxiety; the more items checked, the more severe the anxiety.[6]

How solid were the studies Barlow reviewed? They all claimed to demonstrate that benzodiazepines reduce anxiety. However, when Barlow grouped the studies together to compare the amount of improvement in people who took benzodiazepines to the amount of improvement seen in those who took placebo, he demonstrated that the difference was very slight and could well be accounted for by a change in a single symptom on the Hamilton Scale. In other words, the drugs help with anxiety—but not very much.

Not only were there flaws in many of the articles reviewed by

Barlow, but other studies also have shown little or no benefits to patients when benzodiazepines were prescribed.[7]

The studies by Rickels and Aden and the reviews by Solomon and Barlow looked at the usefulness of benzodiazepines in the treatment of "general" anxiety. By the early eighties, however, panic attacks had been defined as a separate disorder, and researchers began to study these patients. The most famous is the CNCPS funded by Upjohn to promote Xanax.[8] This study involved hundreds of patients and dozens of researchers and played a huge role in refurbishing the reputation of benzodiazepines even before the results of the study were released. Once the results were finally reported, however, numerous deficiencies were apparent.

Washout. There was a washout period of one week prior to patients' enrollment in the study. As noted above, the brevity of this period would bias the results in favor of Xanax. In their review of the marketing of Xanax and the distortions by Upjohn, *Consumer Reports* stated that one investigator refused to participate in the study on the grounds that the brief washout period would automatically bias the study in favor of Xanax.

Dropouts. Many people dropped out of the study before it was finished. About ten percent of the patients on Xanax and fifty percent of those on placebo did not complete the study. The study investigators attributed this to the ineffectiveness of placebo, but there were several other possible explanations.

First, in a different study, 51 out of 119 patients who received diazepam (Valium) dropped out, even though they felt it was effective for anxiety, while there were no dropouts out of 61 patients who were receiving placebo.[9] The dropouts refused further Valium because of negative publicity about it in the press. It is possible that the positive aura around Xanax created by the flow of money and positive information from Upjohn to the doctors in the study contributed to the difference in the dropout rate. Second, the higher dropout rate in the placebo group in the CNCPS could have been due to patients' knowledge that if they dropped out they *would* receive Xanax for their symptoms.[10] This might have led patients to drop out as soon as they realized that they weren't getting Xanax. Third, members of the placebo group may have been experiencing withdrawal symptoms in the first few weeks that those on the Xanax group would have avoided. It is possible that the dropouts' symptoms may have improved over an eight-week period, as most withdrawal symptoms do, if they had stayed in.

Advantage Was Short-lived. The advantage of Xanax over placebo is present only at the end of four weeks. At the end of the full eight weeks of the study there was *no significant difference in the number of panic attacks in those taking Xanax and those taking placebo.*

Upjohn's investigators and marketers emphasized the four-week measurement, which supposedly demonstrates the effectiveness of Xanax, while critics emphasized the eight-week measurement, which supposedly showed its ineffectiveness. The debate over the dropout effect was intense and spilled over into other journals as late as 1993.[11]

Return of symptoms. Patients in the placebo group averaged 2.1 panic attacks after the pills were stopped at the end of the eight-week study. Two weeks later, after the formal end of the study, they averaged only 1.8. Those in the Xanax group averaged 1.7 panic attacks when the pills were stopped at the end of the eight weeks. Within two weeks after the pills were stopped, however, their rate of panic attacks had shot up to 6.8. The return of symptoms only in those who took Xanax clarifies an important point. Whereas the drug suppressed panic attacks only as long as it was taken, people who took placebo derived sustained benefit from their involvement in the study. After the study was concluded, the patients who took placebo were actually better off than those who took Xanax.

Other studies have also found that people experience a return of panic attacks when they stop Xanax and other drugs in this class.[12]

Inadequate Period of Study. Many critics have pointed out that this study, and most others examining the efficacy of benzodiazepiness, examines the effects on patients only for a very short period of time. Panic is clearly a long-term disorder for many people. The average patient in the CNCPS study had been experiencing symptoms for *nine years.* Touting the benefits of a drug that was studied for only eight weeks is somewhat inappropriate and misleading. In a second communication about the CNCPS, Marks pointed out "this study's elephantine labour has resulted in the delivery of a mouse."[13]

The Conclusion of the Report. The abstract of the article mentions only the positive results achieved by Xanax after four weeks. There is no mention that this effect vanished by the time of the eight-week measurement. This significant distortion of the authors' findings inappropriately casts Xanax in a much more favorable light than is warranted.

The Report's Recommendations. In another article reporting the results of the CNCPS, John Pecknold, M.D., who also co-authored the principal report, takes note of the marked increase in panic attacks when patients stop taking Xanax. For this reason, "we recommend that patients with panic disorder be treated for a longer period, at least six months."[14] But even their own data refutes their recommendation. If the effectiveness of Xanax could be demonstrated only at four weeks but not at eight, why would even more time on Xanax be sensible?

As we have seen, the flaws in the study when it was finally published were no match for Upjohn's marketing drive, and Xanax and other benzodiazepines have flourished ever since.

LONG-TERM USAGE STUDIES

Although the vast majority of physicians believe that benzodiazepines are helpful in the short-term management of anxiety, in spite of the flaws in the literature, the use of these drugs for extended periods is a hotly contested issue. Before we look at the arguments, let's look at the few studies that have examined people who have taken benzodiazepines for periods of time longer than just a few weeks.

Most studies have focused on one of three issues. First, do people continue to obtain relief from their anxiety? Second, if they stop taking benzodiazepines do they have a return of any symptoms of anxiety? Third, if they continue to experience anxiety, is this due to the discontinuance syndrome or an ongoing psychiatric disorder? Once again investigators draw different conclusions and give conflicting advice.

Some studies of long-term users appear to demonstrate that benzodiazepines provide continued benefit. One examined twenty-three patients who took diazepam for more than six months, then switched to placebo or stayed on the diazepam. The condition of those in the placebo group worsened. The authors state that this was due not to withdrawal but to the effectiveness of the prior use of diazepam.[15] In an eight-month study comparing alprazolam and imipramine (again funded by Upjohn), alprazolam was found to provide continued benefit for eight months.[16] In a study of neurosurgical patients who had been on diazepam for five years, eighty-three percent reported that they continued to benefit from the medication.[17] A study of twenty-four chronically anxious patients who had been taking diazepam for an average of five years found that symptoms of anxiety gradually returned when it was withdrawn.[18] One study examined 131 patients who had been taking lorazepam or alprazolam for an average of more than three years and concluded that a substantial portion were using their benzodiazepine appropriately for a chronic psychiatric condition.[19] Finally, one study of patients with panic disorder who stayed on alprazolam or clonazepam for more than one year concluded that medication helped but that many patients continued to have residual symptoms that needed additional treatment.[20]

The findings of other studies are somewhat more conflicting. One study examined 180 patients who took diazepam. Fifty percent of the patients had a return of their symptoms when switched to placebo, supposedly demonstrating that diazepam was helpful when taken over a long period of time. However, symptoms did not return in the other fifty percent. An equal number of people, therefore, did just as well when they took a placebo.[21]

In another study, 196 people who had been on diazepam for periods ranging from less than six months to more than ten years were evaluated. Ninety percent had taken the drug for more than six months, seventy-six percent more than two years. The symptoms of patients with long-term usage were the same as those of other patients when they first came for treatment with anxiety. Of the 158 patients who had tried to stop taking diazepam, only 46 reported no emergence of symptoms.[22]

A 1987 study of fifty patients who had taken benzodiazepines from one to twenty-two years and who completed a course of supervised withdrawal found that forty-eight percent were fully recovered and thirty-eight percent were better when evaluated ten months to 3.5 years later. Only six percent were no better, and only eight percent had relapsed.[23]

In 1986 a study was made of 119 long-term users who entered a discontinuation program because they experienced anxiety in spite of their use of benzodiazepines. Many patients had felt unable to stop their medication because of a return of symptoms, and eighty-two percent experienced withdrawal when it was stopped.[24] These findings were replicated in a study by Rickels of fifty-seven other long-term users who attempted to stop their usage. More than half went back on their pills because of continued anxiety. There was one additional intriguing finding, however. Anxiety levels were actually *lower* in the twenty patients who had stopped their pills and were able to stay off them.[25] A continuation of this study confirmed this finding.[26] Rickels performed another study in 1993 on 107 patients given placebo, imipramine, or alprazolam for eight months, tapered over one month and then followed up one year later. No difference in long-term outcome was found between the three groups.[27]

Taken as a group, these studies and others appear to demonstrate that some people who use benzodiazepiness for long periods of time appear to derive some benefit, judging by the return of symptoms of anxiety when an attempt is made to stop the pills. On the other hand, it would appear that some people who take medications actually do worse on them, given that they feel *less* anxious when their drugs are finally stopped. Some patients who experience symptoms of anxiety when their pills are stopped appear to be going through withdrawal, and their symptoms gradually fade away. Others continue to have anxiety and are diagnosed with psychiatric disorders such as panic disorder or depression.

THE EXPERTS DISAGREE

The results of these studies conflict with one another. These conflicts lead different researchers to disagree about the usefulness of benzodiazepines, even when they look at the same data. To understand why this is so it is helpful to look at work by different authors who have reviewed the literature and attempted to reach a sensible conclusion about the wisdom of prolonged use of benzodiazepines.

The American Psychiatric Association convened a task force of more than a dozen psychiatrists to examine the issue. The task force made their report in 1990 in "Benzodiazepine Dependence, Toxicity, and Abuse." The report stated that "controversy regarding risk versus benefits of long-term benzodiazepine use centers around this very point: those who emphasize the therapeutic benefit for the majority of long-term user patients versus those who emphasize the risks of long-term use without clear medical indication and the development of dependence." Carl Salzman, the chairman of the task force, reported in a summary article that the position of the task force was that "the benefits of appropriate theraputic use of benzodiazepines far outweigh the potential risks."[28] They then go on to caution the reader about the importance of trying to avoid dependency. They also state that their "recommendations are generalizations derived from observations from large number of patients and may not apply to a specific clinical situation or to an individual patient. Psychiatrists should always base their prescribing practices on an individual patient's needs rather than on global or general formulations."

This report sends a rather confusing message: The literature review demonstrates that benzodiazepines are reasonable, but generalizations from the literature are not valid for individual patients. One reason for this conflicting message is that it is a consensus document written by many psychiatrists, some of whom have taken opposing stands on the subject from one another in their published work. Second, the report is underwritten by the organization for all psychiatrists. To satisfy all constituencies, therefore, the authors have couched their conclusions in terms that everyone finds tolerable.

In a 170-page supplement to a 1993 issue of *The Journal of Clinical Psychopharmacology* devoted entirely to a comprehensive review of benzodiazepines, Hollister, Oerlinghausen, Rickels, and Shader reviewed 1,400 articles on their usefulness and felt that the short- and long-term use of benzodiazepines was justified.[29] However, they preface their evaluation of benzodiazepines with a description to the reader of what they believe to be five "sources of negative bias" in the literature that obscure the positive effects of benzos:

1. Anxiety is a subjective experience, so that what is recorded depends a great deal on the varying sensibilities of patients and raters.
2. Anxiety disorders are highly variable, and many patients will show relief of anxiety at some point in the course of the disorder even when rating scales show that anxiety is still at appreciable levels. Each patient seems to have a particular threshold of tolerable anxiety.
3. Symptoms of anxiety tend to fade with time. One should

assume that patients enter studies when their levels of anxiety are high, and so some improvement is expected. The beneficial effects of benzodiazepines may be missed or masked by treatment periods so long that spontaneous remission occurs in the patients who take placebo.

4. Patients followed in these studies tend to be those who are regular attendees at clinics, have chronic anxiety reinforced by job, marital, and alcohol problems, and have generally experienced a variety of drugs and some psychotherapy. The investigators state that "it sometimes seems unrealistic to expect them to show measurable responses to a new course of medication."

5. Many studies have too small a sample size to demonstrate that benzodiazepines are more effective.

They summarize their argument by saying: "Considering all these source of negative bias, one can easily see why results of even controlled studies are often disappointing or contradictory. One should be more willing to accept positive results, even when these are incomplete, rather than focus on negative results, which might be artifacts. "Given this method of evaluation, it is not surprising that they recommend the use of benzodiazepines for both short- and long-term usage. In fact, however, their method of analysis stacks the deck *in favor* of benzodiazepines:

1. Why should the subjective nature of anxiety bias the literature *against* benzodiazepines? Many reviewers feel that the subjective nature of the experience of anxiety leads to bias *for* these drugs. People experience many things as helpful for them when they are feeling desperate, even things that are harmful, such as alcohol and drugs. The subjectiveness of the experience of anxiety influences people in both directions.

2. If anxiety disorders are so variable, then the possibility of spontaneous relief would be equally true of people on placebos as for those on medication. In order to demonstrate that benzodiazepines are superior, people on benzodiazepines should still improve at a higher rate than those taking only placeboes. There is no basis for attributing the negative effects of benzos to variability of the illness in adequately controlled studies.

3. If "spontaneous remission" occurs so frequently that the purported positive effects of benzodiazepines can no longer be demonstrated, does this phenomenon in fact indicate "bias" against benzos? The purpose of any study is to see if the drugs help. Finding out that many people don't need that help wouldn't be bias, but a fact.

4. In direct contradiction of the argument in No. 3 that anxiety disorders get better on their own over time, No. 4 argues that people who have chronic anxiety can't be expected to improve with benzos! If we know that it is "unrealistic" for benzos to help people with chronic anxiety, does that reflect a bias in the literature, or is that the answer to the question? It seems almost Orwellian to say that we should prescribe benzodiazepines even though they can't be expected to help.

5. Most studies with inadequate sample size occurred in the fifties, sixties, and seventies. More recent work has not suffered from this deficiency. In fact, though, it was the early work in studies that had too few subjects that supposedly demonstrated the usefulness of benzos, not the other way around.

At least their reasoning to favor benzodiazepines and slant their review of the literature is done in the open, but it is illogical and sabotages the validity of their conclusion that the use of benzodiazepines is justified.

Other experts who review the scientific literature come out against benzodiazepines. For example, English psychiatrist Isaac Marks, author of *Fears, Phobias, and Rituals,* states: "Like all treatments, however, drugs bear a price tag. This includes their cost, the time it takes for them to act, their side effects, the dropout rate, and relapse on stopping drugs . . . the price tag attached to drugs makes them undesirable as the first line treatment."[30]

Marks argues that behavior therapy is more appropriate for anxiety, but he minimizes the problems inherent in behavior therapy research and treatment, slanting his evaluation of the research on benzos. For example, he points to documentation of the effectiveness of behavior therapy as part of his criticism of using benzos. However, he ignores the fact that it is impossible for investigators and the patients to be "blind" to any form of behavior treatment, a standard that he insists be applied to drug treatment research. Also, many patients want relief faster and more easily than can be provided with behavior therapy, factors he dismisses as unimportant. As a clinician who tries to outline all the options for my patients, I know that many people are turned off by a treatment that sounds unfamiliar, difficult, and lengthy. Marks's preference for behavior therapy over benzos may be sensible, but his criticisms of the benzo research are biased because he applies two different standards of proof for evaluation of efficacy.

Norman Miller, an associate professor of psychiatry at the University of Illinois, also criticizes the use of benzodiazepines, this time from the standpoint that they are addictive drugs and as such should be avoided. In a 1995 issue of *Psychiatric Annals* devoted entirely to benzodiazepines, Miller, acting as guest editor, stated that "Despite passionate claims for both sides of the question regarding liability and efficacy involving benzodiazepines, studies are available to form a rational basis for their use in clinical practice . . . [long-term] benzodiazepine-treated patients appeared to be better off and less symptomatic from anxiety and depression when free of benzos."[31]

Miller also slants his review of the literature. He ignores articles that document some benefit to the long-term use of benzodiazepines and cites only Rickels's studies of 1990 and 1993 to substantiate his claim that people are better when they finally stop their benzos. His main concern is that physicians have overlooked the dependence-producing properties of benzos in their rush to treat anxiety. He makes the opposite mistake, however, by ignoring the literature that documents the benefits of benzodiazepines for anxiety and focusing only on their negative qualities.

Clearly, the long-term studies contain contradictions that are not easily understood. Just as clearly, however, one cannot use the conclusion of the short-term studies proving that these drugs can be helpful to minimize anxiety for a few weeks as a guide for whether people should take them for months or years.

THE CAUSE OF THE CONTRADICTIONS

I have highlighted some of the contradictions in the literature to demonstrate that there is no clear message about the efficacy of long-term benzodiazepine use. Different researchers reach very different conclusions about data from the same studies. What can we salvage from this mass of confusion? Is there anything of value here, or are all the scientists too biased and the data too confusing? Are there factors in the studies of anxiety and benzodiazepines that have not been focused on that could lead to different findings in different studies?

I believe that the answer is most definitely yes. A number of factors, many of them only minimally explored, influence the results of these studies in a profound way. After we look at some of those factors, the reason for contradictory findings will be clear.

The Effect of Hope

In the CNCPS, sixty-seven percent of patients suffering from spontaneous panic attacks (i.e., panic attacks that are not caused by exposure to a specific object or environment, such as a supermarket) who were given a placebo and who finished the study had a full resolution of the attacks. This is a very high percentage. Although the study does show that Xanax is also effective—eighty-one percent of patients who received it also had resolution—sixty-seven percent is still pretty good for a sugar pill. The usual rate of improvement of patients who take placebo in other psychiatric drug studies is about one-third.

Placebos didn't help patients with strep throats, measles, or broken legs. Anxiety is different because it can be affected so strongly by a person's hope. The effectiveness of the measles vaccine, for instance, is not influenced by whether one hopes or expects that it works. The large positive effect on anxiety obtained by people in the CNCPS taking a placebo is unusual for any disorder. It makes the validity of any study of anxiety questionable because so many factors can affect a person's hopefulness. These include religious beliefs, the encouragement of friends and family, or even the participation in a study at all.

The Effect of Patients' Knowledge

As we have noted, the CNCPS experienced dropouts in the placebo group, while another study noted that all fifty-one dropouts in a comparison study of the effects of diazepam and placebo were in the diazepam group.[32] Sixty-three percent of the patients in the diazepam study relapsed and sought medical or psychiatric care within a year after the study was terminated.[33] One half of the people who relapsed did not restart diazepam in spite of the fact that it had been previously effective for them. The dropouts' refusal to go back on the drug was due to the heightened publicity about its negative effects.

Let's think about this for a moment. Imagine that you had intense anxiety and that you were recruited for a study to take a new drug that might be helpful for the treatment of anxiety. Now imagine that you were recruited for a study to take a drug you heard through the media was addictive and potentially harmful. Hearing two such different messages can set up very different expectations, in spite of the fact that the drugs are virtually equivalent in their therapeutic effects and the tendency to cause dependence. Clearly this information would change your attitude about taking the drug and completing the study.

The difference in dropout rates demonstrates that attitudes toward benzodiazepines can significantly influence a person's behavior and willingness to take them and may substantially alter the results of a study.

The Effect of Doctors' Visits

In their letter criticizing the conclusions of the investigators of the CNCPS, Marks and his co-authors focused on the high rate of placebo response.[34] They hypothesized that perhaps these people were helped by the regular (weekly) trips in which they saw a doctor.

Most of us feel that we have an ally when we meet with our doctor. This can have a positive effect on the course of any illness, whether medical, surgical, or psychiatric. In the CNCPS, the patients met with a doctor every week to review their symptoms and to get their medicine. It is likely that this consistent attention would have a powerful effect above and beyond that of the medicine.

Other investigators who have followed patients after the formal end of their studies in which benzodiazepines were used have also found that many patients have relapsed. One has to ask whether the initial improvement shown in the CNCPS was due to the medicine or to regular contact with a physician. The CNCPS did not take this factor into account.

The Effect of Exposure to an Anxiety-Provoking Situation

As Joseph Wolpe, world-reknowned researcher into anxiety and behavior therapy, described in 1973 in *The Practice of Behavior Therapy*, exposure to an anxiety-provoking situation can help people overcome their usual symptoms of anxiety. Marks, an advocate of behavior therapy, points out that patients may have benefited from the weekly trips to see the doctors involved in the study. Simply by participating in the study, the patients exposed themselves to situations that they normally avoided, such as leaving their house. Was improvement at eight weeks for patients taking placebo or Xanax actually due to this factor and not to the pills at all?

The Effect of Inadvertent and Deliberate Distortion by Patients

Another factor that causes different studies to reach different conclusions is the difficulty of getting reliable answers from the study's patients. In many of these studies a problem has emerged that must be taken into account: Some subjects take benzodiazepines that they have obtained elsewhere and don't tell the researchers. This only became apparent when researchers started to draw blood levels of the medications on patients they were studying in order to understand more clearly the relationship of dosage size, drug blood level, and clinical response. In order to maintain strict adherence to a double-blind protocol, researchers drew blood on all patients, those taking the benzodiazepine and those actually receiving placebo. Researchers found that benzodiazepines were occasionally in the blood of some of the people who were taking placebo. This could potentially affect the validity of a study if enough people in the placebo group took medication surreptitiously.

Because of this, current investigators draw blood on all subjects to measure the presence of drugs. One study found that eight percent (four in forty-eight) were taking benzodiazepines from another source without telling investigators.[35] How reliable are results when study subjects actively lie about their drug use? Perhaps they are also misrepresenting their use of other drugs, or even exaggerating their symptoms in order to get the drugs. The validity of any study is open to question when patients lie about such important factors.

The Effect of a Patient's Perception of Anxiety

Although researchers sometimes measure the intensity or severity of a patient's symptoms, they rarely describe the meaning of those symptoms to the patient who has them. Some people with anxiety think that their symptoms are troubling and want help with them until they get their lives back on track, while other patients with similar symptoms wonder if they are going crazy, think that they must be having a nervous breakdown, and may even want to be in a psychiatric hospital for safety. These very different patient perceptions of what anxiety means would obviously influence anyone's experience of medication. Many people who were able to get their life back on track to some extent and who stay on benzodiazepines primarily to avoid the symptoms of withdrawal might very well experience less anxiety when they finally got off their drug. This might account for some researchers finding that anxiety levels were lower for some people after they stopped their drug. On the other hand, people who were overwhelmed by their anxiety might very well find their symptoms worse when their medication is stopped.

The Effect of Different Stresses Leading to Anxiety

Different stresses in a person's life can lead to a very different experience of anxiety. Sexual abuse by a father is quite different from the death of a mother, but both can lead to panic attacks, panic disorder, and chronic benzodiazepine use. Someone who restricted herself to home because of chronic fearfulness due in part to the premature death of a mother might find weekly visits to an authority figure like an investigator helpful and find that she gets better as the study proceeds. On the other hand, someone who stays at home because severe sexual abuse in her past made her fearful of men might find weekly visits to male authority figures very anxiety provoking and might demonstrate no improvement in her symptoms of anxiety.

CONCLUSION

Studies contradict one another and different reviewers provide varying interpretations of the results. On a superficial level, the conflicts are due to the specific limitations of each study and the biases of different reviewers. On a deeper level, however, it is the complex and subjective nature of anxiety itself that leads to the contradictions. The constellation of a person's genetic and biological makeup, his early experiences in life, his thoughts, feelings, sensations, and behaviors manifesting his anxiety, and the way that he copes with anxiety is unique to each individual. Although the *sensations* of anxiety are similar in different people, no two people have the same overall experience of anxiety. No investigator can adequately control for the myriad factors that constitute the total process of a person's anxiety. As a result, each study discovers its own "truth." Taken as a whole, therefore, the literature provides no valid guidance about the value of the long-term usefulness of benzodiazepines for a person with chronic anxiety.

The destructive influence of benzodiazepines and the need for more effective treatment becomes clear only with a close examination of all aspects of a person's life. This is a task that best takes place between a doctor and a patient, not an investigator and a subject.

NOTES

CHAPTER 1

1. *APA Task Force Report* 1990.
2. Hollister 1961.
3. Lader 1983a, 1983b, 1983c, 1984a, 1987, 1991.
4. Mellinger 1984a, Mellinger 1984b, Rodrigo 1988, Salzman 1993.
5. Balter 1984, Busto 1996.
6. Ashton 1989, Dunbar 1989, *APA Task Force Report* 1990.

CHAPTER 2

1. *DSM-IV.* The *DSM-IV* is published by the American Psychiatric Association and contains specific criteria necessary to differentiate one psychiatric diagnosis from another. It is the standard manual used by most professionals in the field to diagnose their patients and justify their treatment recommendations to the patients and to any third-party payers.
2. Noyes 1990.
3. Kessler 1994.
4. Ibid.
5. Fava 1988.
6. Kessler 1994.
7. Ibid.
8. Gordon 1979.
9. Mellinger 1984a.
10. Burke 1995.

CHAPTER 3

1. Sheehan 1983.
2. Kagan 1984.
3. Crowe, 1983, Rosenbaum 1988, Last 1991, Rosenbaum 1992, Skre 1994, Kendler 1995, Silove 1995.
4. Torgerson 1983.
5. Crowe 1983, Last 1991, Rosenbaum 1992.
6. Crowe 1980.
7. Mazza 1988.
8. Clark 1982, 1986.
9. Clark 1985.
10. Rainey 1987, Southwick 1993.

11. Kaplan and Sadock 1981.
12. Beck 1992, Otto 1992, 1994, Spiegel 1994, Bruce 1995.
13. van der Kolk 1984, 1987, 1988, 1996; Herman 1992.
14. Taylor and Arnow 1988.
15. van der Kolk 1985, 1987, 1988, 1989, Pitman 1990.
16. Bremner 1995.

CHAPTER 4
1. Mohler 1978, Paul 1979, Tallman 1980, Snyder 1981, Lader 1987.
2. Hollister 1961, Petursson 1981, Lader 1983a, 1983c, 1984a, 1987, 1991, Schopf 1983, Marks, J. 1983, Haskell 1986, Noyes 1988, Rickels 1988, Roy-Byrne 1989, Noyes 1991, Ashton 1991a.
3. Lader 1983b, Ladewig 1984, Rickels 1986b, Lin 1989.
4. *APA Task Force Report* 1990.
5. Schweizer 1990.
6. Goodman 1990.
7. Lader 1991.
8. *New York Times,* 11/6/79, p. A18.
9. Lader 1978.
10. Rickels 1983.
11. Klerman 1988.
12. Ballenger 1989.
13. Breggin 1991.
14. *Consumer Reports* 1993.
15. Catalan 1985, Lader 1993, Ashton 1994.
16. Weintraub 1991, Reidenberg 1991, McNutt 1994.
17. Brahams 1990.
18. Sheehan 1983.
19. Miller 1991, *APA Task Force Report* 1990.
20. Raft 1975.
21. Gullick 1979.
22. Wolpe 1973, Marks 1987, Gelernter 1991, de Beurs 1995.
23. McClusky 1991.
24. *Wall Street Journal* 12/1/95, p. 1.
25. Bartels 1997.

CHAPTER 5
1. Barlow 1988.
2. Faravelli 1985, Roy-Byrne 1986, Shore 1986, Breslau 1991, van der Kolk 1984, 1987, 1988, 1996, Herman 1992, Wallerstein 1989, Bryer 1987.
3. Kendler 1992.
4. Russell 1984.
5. Browne 1986, Bryer 1987, Herman 1986, 1989, 1992, Stein 1996, Pribor 1992, Fierman 1993.
6. Brady 1981.
7. Kritsberg 1985.

8. Webb 1992.
9. Post 1991
10. Black 1982.
11. Ibid.
12. Wallerstein 1980.
13. Wallerstein 1989.
14. Herman 1986, van der Kolk 1984, 1991, Lee 1995.

CHAPTER 6

1. Mellinger 1984, Balter 1984, *APA Task Force Report* 1990, Summers 1990, Ashton 1991b.
2. Schatzberg 1991.
3. Kessler 1994.
4. Kagan 1984.
5. Ainsworth 1978.
6. Shore 1986, Palinkas 1993.
7. Breslau 1991.
8. Herman 1981.
9. Gilligan 1982.
10. Miller 1976.
11. Jordan 1991.
12. Ettore 1994.
13. Kessler 1994.
14. Ettore 1994.
15. *DSM-IV.*
16. Horwitz 1977.
17. Anderson 1981.
18. Weyerer 1991.
19. Ettore 1994.
20. Ettore 1987.
21. Frankfort 1972, Boston Women's Health Collective 1976, Ehrenreich 1978.
22. *Life* 1956 41 (26) p. 115.
23. Morabia 1992.
24. Maccoby 1974, Block 1984, Lipman-Blumen 1984, Prather 1991, Ettore 1987.
25. Ettore 1994.
26. Balint 1969.

CHAPTER 7

1. Woods 1987, Simpson 1990, Thompson 1995, *APA Task Force Report* 1990.
2. Cook 1983, Pomara 1985, Nikaido 1987.
3. *PDR* 1996.
4. Cook 1983, Pomara 1985.
5. *PDR* 1996.
6. Curren 1987.

7. *APA Task Force Report* 1990.
8. *PDR* 1996.
9. Ashton 1995.
10. Gardner 1985.
11. *PDR* 1996.
12. Woods 1987, *APA Task Force Report* 1990.
13. Kales 1973, Kales, 1978.
14. Ashton 1995.
15. Ibid.
16. Hendler 1980.
17. Golombok 1988.
18. Lader 1984b.
19. Schmauss 1987.
20. Uhdi 1987.
21. Poser 1983.
22. Perera 1987.
23. Andreasen 1990.
24. Moodley 1993.
25. Ashton 1995.
26. Laegrid 1990.
27. Altshuler 1996.
28. Bergman 1992.
29. Cummings 1985, Melton 1983, Tinetti 1988.
30. Tinetti 1988.
31. Macdonald 1985.
32. Ray 1987.
33. Tinetti 1988.
34. Campbell 1989.
35. Gales 1995.
36. *APA Task Force Report* 1990.
37. Oster 1990.
38. Neutel 1995.
39. Ray 1992.
40. Serfaty 1993.
41. Melander 1991.
42. Brahams 1990.
43. Lader 1983a, *APA Task Force Report* 1990.
44. Busto 1983, Wiseman 1985, Ross 1993.
45. *APA Task Force Report* 1990.
46. Ashton 1995.

CHAPTER 8
1. *APA Task Force Report* 1990.
2. Herz 1992, Herz 1993.
3. Lader 1993.
4. Morrice 1990.
5. Gillin 1991.

6. Schneider-Helmert 1988.
7. Gillin 1991.
8. McClusky 1991, Milby, 1993.

CHAPTER 9
1. Benson 1975.
2. Miller 1969.
3. Wolpe 1973, Mavissakalian 1986, Marks 1987, Ost 1989, Gelernter 1991, de Beurs 1995.
4. Beck 1985, 1992, Otto 1992, 1993, 1994, Spiegel 1994, Bruce 1995.
5. Milrod 1991a, 1991b, 1995, 1996, Shear 1993.

CHAPTER 10
1. Cormack 1989.

CHAPTER 11
1. Clum 1990.

CHAPTER 12
1. Ross 1993.
2. Ciraulo 1988.
3. Serfaty 1993.

APPENDIX
1. Jenner 1961, Azima 1962, Daneman 1964, Tobin 1964, Chesrow 1965.
2. Rickels 1967.
3. Solomon 1978.
4. Aden 1980.
5. Barlow 1988.
6. Hamilton 1959.
7. Shapiro 1983, Catalan 1984a, Catalan 1984b, Caplan 1985, Tyrer 1988.
8. Ballenger 1988, Pecknold 1988.
9. Rickels 1983.
10. Marks 1989.
11. *Consumer Reports* 1993.
12. Fyer 1987.
13. Marks 1992.
14. Pecknold 1988.
15. Bowden 1980.
16. Schweizer 1993.
17. Hollister 1981.
18. Laughren 1982.
19. Romach 1995.
20. Pollack 1993.

21. Rickels 1983.
22. Haskell 1986.
23. Ashton 1987.
24. Rickels 1986a.
25. Rickels 1990.
26. Rickels 1991.
27. Rickels 1993.
28. *APA Task Force Report* 1990.
29. Hollister 1993.
30. Marks 1987.
31. Miller 1995.
32. Rickels 1983.
33. Rickels 1984.
34. Marks 1989.
35. Rickels 1993.

BIBLIOGRAPHY

Aden, G. C., and Thein, S. G. Alprazolam Compared to Diazepam and Placebo in the Treatment of Anxiety. *Journal of Clinical Anxiety* 1980; 41:245–248.

Ainsworth, M. D. S., Blehar, M. C., Waters, E., and Wall, S. *Patterns of Attachment: A Psychological Study of the Strange Situation.* Lawrence Erlbaum Associates Inc., 1978 Hillsdale, New Jersey.

Altshuler, L. L., Cohen, L., Szuba, M. P., Burt, V. K., Gitlin, M., Mintz, J. Pharmacological Management of Psychiatric Illness During Pregnancy: Dilemmas and Guidelines. *American Journal of Psychiatry* 1996; 153:592–606.

American Psychiatric Association. *Diagnostic and Statistical Manual of Mental Disorders (DSM-IV).* American Psychiatric Association, 1994, Washington, D.C.

American Psychiatric Association Task Force Report. *Benzodiazepine: Dependence, Toxicity and Abuse.* American Psychiatric Association, 1990, Washington, D.C.

Anderson, J. E. Prescribing of Tranquilizers to Women and Men. *Canadian Medical Association Journal* 1981; 125:1229–1232.

Andreasen, N. C., Swayze II, V., Flaum, M., Alliger, R., Cohen, G. Ventricular Abnormalities in Affective Disorder: Clinical and Demographic Correlates. *American Journal of Psychiatry* 1990; 147:893–900.

Ashton, H. Benzodiazepine Withdrawal: Outcome in 50 Patients. *British Journal of Addiction* 1987; 82: 665–671.

———. Protracted Withdrawal Syndromes from Benzodiazepines. *Journal of Substance Abuse Treatment* 1991a; 8:19–28.

———. Psychotropic-Drug Prescribing for Women. *British Journal of Psychiatry* 1991b; 158 (supplement 10): 30–35.

———. Guidelines for the Rational Use of Benzodiazepines. When and What to Use. *Drugs* 1994; 48(1):25–40.

———. Toxicity and Adverse Consequences of Benzodiazepine Use. *Psychiatric Annals* 1995; 25(3):158–165.

Ashton, H., and Golding, J. F. Tranquillisers: Prevalence, Predictors and Possible Consequences. Data from a large United Kingdom survey. *British Journal of Addiction* 1989; 84:541–546.

Azima, H., Arthurs, D., and Silver, A. The Effects of Chlordiazepoxide (Librium) in Anxiety States. A Multi-Blind Study. *Canadian Psychiatric Association Journal* 1962; 7:44–50.

Balint, M. *The Basic Fault.* Tavistock Publications 1969 London.

Ballenger, J. C., Burrows, G. D., DuPont, R. L., Lesser, I. M., Noyes Jr., R. Pecknold, J. C., Rifkin, A., and Swinson, R. P. Alprazolam in Panic Disorder and Agoraphobia: Results from a Multicenter Trial. I. Efficacy in Short-term Treatment. *Archives of General Psychiatry* 1988; 45:413–422.

Balter, M. B., Manheimer, D. I., Mellinger, G. D., and Uhlenhuth, E. H. A Cross-National Comparison of Anti-Anxiety/Sedative Drug Use. *Current Medical Research and Opinion* 1984; 8 (supplement 4):5–20.

Barlow, D. H. *Anxiety and Its Disorders: The Nature and Treatment of Anxiety and Panic.* The Guilford Press 1988 New York.

Bartels, S., Horn, S., Sharkey, P., Mental Health Services and Elderly Primary Care Patients in HMOs: Results From the Managed Care Outcomes Project. Presented at the annual meeting of the American Association of Geriatric Psychiatry February 1997.

Beck, A. T., Sokol, L., Clark, D. A., Berchick, R., and Wright, F. A Crossover Study of Focused Cognitive Therapy for Panic Disorder. *American Journal of Psychiatry* 1992; 149:778–783.

Beck, A. T., and Emery, G., with Greenberg, R. L. *Anxiety Disorders and Phobias: A Cognitive Perspective.* Basic Books 1985 New York.

Benson, H. *The Relaxation Response.* Avon Books 1975 New York.

Bergman, U., Rosa, F. W., Baum, C., Wiholm B. E., and Faich, G. A. Effects of Exposure to Benzodiazepine During Fetal Life. *Lancet* 1992; 340:694–696.

de Beurs, E., van Balkom, A. J. L. M., Lange, A., Koele, P., van Dyck, R. Treatment of Panic Disorder with Agoraphobia: Comparison of Fluvoxamine, Placebo, and Psychological Panic Management Combined with Exposure and of Exposure in Vivo Alone. *American Journal of Psychiatry* 1995; 152:683–691.

Black, C. B., *It Will Never Happen to Me.* M. A. C. 1982 Denver, Colorado.

Block, J. *Sex-Role Identity and Ego Development.* Jossey-Bass 1984 San Francisco.

Boston Women's Health Collective. *Our Bodies, Our Selves.* Simon & Schuster 1976 New York.

Bowden, C. L., and Fisher, J. G. Safety and Efficacy of Long-Term Diazepam Therapy. *Southern Medical Journal* 1980 73(12):1581–1584.

Brady, K. *Father's Days: A True Story of Incest.* Dell Publishing Co. Inc. 1981 New York.

Brahams, D. Benzodiazepine Overprescribing: Successful Initiative in New York State. *Lancet* Dec. 1, 1990; 336:1372–1373.

Breggin, P. R. *Toxic Psychiatry.* St. Martin's Press 1991 New York.

Bremner, J. D., Randall, P., Scott, T., Bronen, R. A., Seibyl, J. P., Southwick, S. M., Delaney, R. C., McCarthy, G., Charney, D. S., and Innis, R. B. MRI-Based Measurement of Hippocampal Volume in Patients with Combat-Related Posttraumatic Stress Disorder. *American Journal of Psychiatry* 1995; 152(7):973–981.

Breslau, N., Davis, G. C., Andreski, P., Peterson, E. Traumatic Events and Posttraumatic Stress Disorder in an Urban Population of Young Adults. *Archives of General Psychiatry* 1991; 48:216-222.

Browne, A., and Finkelhor, D. Impact of Child Sexual Abuse: A Review of the Research. *Psychological Bulletin* 1986; 99(1):66–77.

Bruce, T. J., Spiegel, D. A., Gregg, S. F., and Nuzzarello, A. Predictors of Alprazolam Discontinuation With and Without Cognitive Behavior Therapy in Panic Disorder. *American Journal of Psychiatry* 1995; 152:1156–1160.

Bryer, J. B., Nelson, B. A., Miller, J. B., and Krol, P. A. Childhood Sexual and Physical Abuse as Factors in Adult Psychiatric Illness. *American Journal of Psychiatry* 1987; 144:1426–1430.

Burke, K. C., Meek, W. J., Krych, R., Nisbet, R., Burke, J. D. Medical Services Use by Patients Before and After Detoxification from Benzodiazepine Dependence. *Psychiatric Services* 1995; 46(2):157–160.

Buster, U., Ruiz, I., Busto, M., Gactiva, A. Benzodiazepine Use in Chile: Impact of Availability on Use, Abuse, and Dependence. *Journal of Clinical Psychopharmacology* 1996; 16:363–72.

Busto, U., Simpkins, J., Sellers, E. M., Sisson, B., and Segal, R. Objective Determination of Benzodiazepine Use and Abuse in Alcoholics. *British Journal of Addiction* 1983; 78:429–435.

Campbell, A. J., Borrie, M. J., and Spears, G. F. Risk Factors for Falls in a Community-Based Prospective Study of People 70 Years and Older. *Journal of Gerontology: Medical Sciences* 1989; 44:M112-117.

Caplan, R. D., Andrews, F. M., Conway, T. L., Abbey, A., Abramis, D. J., and French Jr., J. R. P. Social Effects of Diazepam Use: A Longitudinal Field Study. *Social Science and Medicine* 1985; 21(8):887–898.

Catalan, J., Gath, D. H., Benzodiazepines in General Practice: Time for a Decision. *British Medical Journal.* 1985; 290:1374–1376.

Catalan, J., Gath, D. H., Edmonds, G., and Ennis, J. The Effects of Non-Prescribing of Anxiolytics in General Practice: I. Controlled Evaluation of Psychiatric and Social Outcome. *British Journal of Psychiatry* 1984; 144:593–602.

Catalan, J., Gath, D. H., Bond, A., and Martin, P. The Effects of Non-Prescribing of Anxiolytics in General Practice: II. Factors Associated with Outcome. *British Journal of Psychiatry* 1984; 144:603–610.

Chesrow, E. J., Kaplitz, S. E., Vetra, H., et al. Blind Study of Oxazepam for the Management of Geriatric Patients with Behavioral Problems. *Clinical Medicine* 1965; 72:1001–1005.

Ciraulo, D. A., Barnhill, J. G., Greenblatt, D. J., Shader, R. I., Ciraulo, A. M., Tarmey, M. F., Molloy, M. A., and Foti, M. E. Abuse Liability and Clinical Pharmacokinetics of Alprazolam in Alcoholic Men. *Journal of Clinical Psychiatry* 1988; 49:333–337.

Clark, D. M., and Hemsley, D. R. The Effects of Hyperventilation; Individual Variability and its Relation to Personality. *Journal of Behavior Therapy and Experimental Psychiatry* 1982; 13(1):41-47.

Clark, D. A Cognitive Approach to Panic. *Behaviour Research and Therapy* 1986; 24(4):461–470.

Clark, D., Salkovskis, P. M., and Chalkley, A. J. Respiratory Control As a Treatment for Panic Attacks. *Journal of Behavior Therapy and Experimental Psychiatry* 1985: 16(1):23–30.

Clum, G. A. *Coping with Panic: A Drug-Free Approach to Dealing with Panic Attacks.* Brooks/Cole Publishing Company 1990 Belmont, California.

Consumer Reports. High Anxiety. January 1993; 19–24

Cook, P. J., Huggett, A., Graham-Pole, R., Savage, I. T., and James, I. M. Hypnotic Accumulation and Hangover in Elderly Inpatients: A Controlled Double-Blind Study of Temazepam and Nitrazepam. *British Medical Journal* 1983; 286:100–102.

Cormack, M. A., Owens, R. G., and Dewey, M. E. The Effect of Minimal Interventions by General Practitioners on Long-Term Benzodiazepine Use. *Journal of the Royal College of General Practitioners* 1989; 39:408–411.

Crowe, R. R., Pauls, D. L., Slymen, D. J., Noyes, R. A Family Study of Anxiety Neurosis. *Archives of General Psychiatry* 1980; 37:77–79.

Crowe, R. R., Noyes, R., Pauls, D. L., Slymen, D. A Family Study of Panic Disorder. *Archives of General Psychiatry* 1983; 40:1065–1069.

Cummings, S. R., Kelsey, J. L., Nevitt, M. C., O'Dowd, K. J. Epidemiology of Osteoporosis and Osteoporotic Fractures. *Epidemiologic Review* 1985; 7:178–208.

Curran, H. V., Schiwy, W., and Lader, M. Differential Amnesic Properties of Benzodiazepines: A Dose-Response Comparison of Two Drugs with Similar Elimination Half-lives. *Psychopharmacology* 1987; 92:358–364.

Daneman, F. A. Double-Blind Study with Diazepam, Chlordiazepoxide and Placebo in the Treatment of Psychoneurotic Anxiety. *J Med Assoc GA* 1964 53:55–58.

Dunbar, G. C., Perera, M. H., and Jenner, F. A. Patterns of Benzodiazepine Use in Great Britain. *British Journal of Psychiatry* 1989; 155:836–841.

Ehrenreich, B., and English, D. *For Her Own Good: 150 Years of the Experts' Advice to Women.* Anchor Books Edition 1979 Garden City, New York.

Ettorre, E. *Women and Substance Use.* Rutgers University Press 1987 Princeton, NJ.

Ettorre, E., Klaukka, T., and Riska, E. Psychotropic Drugs: Long-Term Use, Dependency and the Gender Factor. *Social Science Medicine* 1994 39(12):1667–1673.

Faravelli, C., Webb, T., Ambonetti, A., Fonnesu, F., and Sessarego, A. Prevalence of Traumatic Early Life Events in 31 Agoraphobic Patients with Panic Attacks. *American Journal of Psychiatry* 1985; 142:1493–1494.

Fava, G. A., Grandi, S., Canestrari, R. Prodromal Symptoms in Panic Disorder with Agoraphobia. *American Journal of Psychiatry* 1988; 145:1564–1567.

Fierman, E. J., Hunt, M. F., Pratt, L. A., Warshaw, M. G., Yonkers, K. A., Peterson, L. G., Epstein-Kaye, T. M., Norton, H. S. Trauma and Post-traumatic Stress Disorder in Subjects with Anxiety Disorders. *American Journal of Psychiatry* 1993; 150:1872–1874

Frankfurt, E. *Vaginal Politics.* Quadrangle Press 1976 New York.

Fyer, A. J., Liebowitz, M. R., Gorman, J. M., Campeas, R., Levin, A., Davies, S. O., Goetz, D., Klein, D. F. Discontinuation of Alprazolam Treatment in Panic Patients. *American Journal of Psychiatry* 1987; 144:303–308.

Gales, B. J., and Menard, S. M. Relationship Between the Administration of Selected Medications and Falls in Hospitalized Elderly Patients. *Annals of Pharmacotherapy* 1995; 29:354–358.

Gardner, D. L., and Cowdry, R. W. Alprazolam-Induced Dyscontrol in Borderline Personality Disorder. *American Journal of Psychiatry* 1985; 142:98–100.

Gelernter, C. S., Uhde, T. W., Cimbolic, P., Arnkoff, D. B., Vittone, B. J., Tancer, M. E., Bartko, J. J. Cognitive-Behavioral and Pharmacological Treatments of Social Phobia: A Controlled Study. *Archives of General Psychiatry* 1991; 48:939–945.

Gilligan, C. *In a Different Voice.* Harvard University Press 1982 Cambridge, Mass.

Gillin, J. C. The Long and the Short of Sleeping Pills. *New England Journal of Medicine* 1991; 324(24):1735–1737.

Golombok, S., Moodley, P., and Lader, M. Cognitive Impairment in Long-Term Benzodiazepine Users. *Psychological Medicine* 1988; 18:365–374.

Goodman, G. A., Rall, T. W., Nies, A. S., and Taylor, P. *Goodman and Gilman's The Pharmacological Basis of Therapeutics.* Pergamon Press 1990 New York.

Gordon, B. *I'm Dancing As Fast As I Can.* Harper and Row 1979 New York.

Gullick, E. L., and King, L. J. Appropriateness of Drugs Prescribed by Primary Care Physicians for Depressed Outpatients. *Journal of Affective Disorders* 1979; 1:55–58.

Hamilton, M. The Assessment of Anxiety States by Rating. *Journal of Medical Psychology* 1959; 32:50–55.

Haskell, D., Cole, J. O., Schniebolk, S., and Lieberman, B. A Survey of Diazepam Patients. *Psychopharmacology Bulletin* 1986; 22(2)434–438.

Hendler, N., Cimini, C., Ma, T., and Long, D. A Comparison of Cognitive Impairment Due to Benzodiazepines and to Narcotics. *American Journal of Psychiatry* 1980; 137(7):828–830.

Herman, J. L. *Father-Daughter Incest.* Harvard University Press 1981 Cambridge, Mass.

———. *Trauma and Recovery.* Basic Books 1992 New York.

Herman, J. L., Perry, J. C., van der Kolk, B. A. Childhood Trauma in Borderline Personality Disorder. *American Journal of Psychiatry* 1989; 146(4) 490–495.

Herman, J. L., Russell, D., Trocki, K. Long-Term Effects of Incestuous Abuse in Childhood. *American Journal of Psychiatry* 1986; 143(10):1293–1296.

Herz, M. A Benzodiazepine Sketch of a War. *Family Medicine* 1992; 24(6):411–412.

———. Benzodiazepine Prescribing in a Community in Crisis. *Family Practice* 1993; 10(3):317–319.

Hollister, L. E., Conley, F. K., Britt, R. H., and Sheur, L. Long-term Use of Diazepam. *Journal of the American Medical Association* 1981; 246:1568–1570.

Hollister, L. E., Motzenbecker, F. P., Degen, R. O. Withdrawal Reactions from Chlordiazepoxide (Librium). *Psychopharmacologia* 1961; 2:63–68.

Hollister, L. E., Muller-Oerlinghausen, B., Rickels, K., and Shader, R. I. Clinical Uses of Benzodiazepines. *Journal of Clinical Psychopharmacology* 1993; 13(6)(supplement 1):1S–169S.

Horwitz, A. The Pathways into Psychiatric Treatment: Some Differences Between Men and Women. *Journal of Health and Social Policy* 1977; 18:169–178.

Hughes, R., and Brewin, R. *The Tranquilizing of America: Pill-popping and the American Way of Life.* Harcourt Bruce 1979 San Diego.

Jenner, F. A., Keery, R. J., and Parkin, D. A Controlled Trial of Methaminodiazepoxide (Chlordiazepoxide, "Librium") in the Treatment of Anxiety in Neurotic Patients. *Journal of Mental Science* 1961; 107:575–582.

Jordan, J. V., Kaplan, A. G., Miller, J. B., Stiver, I. P., and Surrey, J. L. *Women's Growth in Connection: Writings from the Stone Center.* The Guilford Press 1991 New York.

Kagan, J. *The Nature of the Child.* Basic Books 1984 New York.

Kales, A., Bixler, E. O., Kales, J. D., and Scharf, M. B. Comparative Effectiveness of Nine Hypnotic Drugs: Sleep Laboratory Studies. *Journal of Clinical Pharmacology* 1977; 17(4):207–213.

Kales, A., and Kales, J. D. Sleep Laboratory Studies of Hypnotic Drugs: Efficacy and Withdrawal Effects. *Journal of Clinical Psychopharmacology* 1983; 3(2):140–150.

Kaplan, H. I., Sadock, B. J. *Modern Synopsis of Comprehensive Textbook of Psychiatry/IV.* Williams and Wilkins 1985 Baltimore.

Kendler, K. S., Neale, M. C., Kessler, R. C., Heath, A. C., and Eaves, L. J. Childhood Parental Loss and Adult Psychopathology in Women. A Twin Study Perspective. *Archives of General Psychiatry* 1992; 49:109–116.

Kendler, K. S., Walters, E. E., Neale, M. C., Kessler, R. C., Heath, A. C., and Eaves, L. J. The Structure of the Genetic and Environmental Risk Factors for Six Major Psychiatric Disorders in Women. *Archives of General Psychiatry* 1995; 52:374–383.

Kessler, R. C., McGonagle, K. A., Zhao, S., Nelson, C. B., Hughes, M., Eshleman, S., Wittchin, H. U., and Kendler, K. S. Lifetime and 12-Month Prevalence of DSM-III-R Psychiatric Disorders in the United States. *Archives of General Psychiatry* 1994; 51:8–19.

Klerman, G. L. Overview of the Cross-National Collaborative Panic Study. *Archives of General Psychiatry* 1988; 45:407–412.

van der Kolk, B. A. *Psychological Trauma.* American Psychiatric Press 1987 Washington, D.C.

———. The Trauma Spectrum: the Interaction of Biological and Social Events in the Genesis of the Trauma Response. *Journal of Traumatic Stress* 1988; 1:273–290.

van der Kolk, B. A., Blitz, R., Burr, W., Sherry, S., Hartmann, E. Nightmares and Trauma: A Comparison of Nightmares After Combat with Lifelong Nightmares in Veterans. *American Journal of Psychiatry* 1984; 141(2) 187–190.

van der Kolk, B. A., Greenberg, M. S., Boyd, H., Krystal, J. Inescapable Shock, Neurotransmitters and Addiction to Trauma: Towards a Psychobiology of Post Traumatic Stress. *Biological Psychiatry* 1985; 20:314–325.

van der Kolk, B. A., Greenberg, M. S., Orr, S. P., Pitman, R. K. Endogenous Opioids, Stress-Induced Analgesia, and Post-Traumatic Stress Disorder. *Psychopharmacology Bulletin* 1989; 25:417–421.

van der Kolk, B. A., McFarlane, M. C., Weisaeth, L. *Traumatic Stress: The Effects of Overwhelming Experience on Mind, Body, and Society.* Guilford Press 1996 New York.

van der Kolk, B. A., Perry, J. C., Herman, J. L. Childhood Origins of Self-Destructive Behavior. *American Journal of Psychiatry* 1991; 148(12)1665–1671.

Kritsberg, W. *The Adult Children of Alcoholics Syndrome.* Health Communications Inc. 1985 Pompano Beach, Fla.

Lader, M. Benzodiazepines—The Opium of the Masses? *Neuroscience* 1978; 3:159–165.

———. Dependence on Benzodiazepines. *Journal of Clinical Psychiatry* 1983a; 44:121–127.

———. Benzodiazepine Dependence. *Progress in Neuro-Psychopharmacology and Biological Psychiatry* 1984a; 8:85–95.

———. The Biological Basis of Benzodiazepine Dependence. *Psychological Medicine* 1987; 17:539–547.

———. History of Benzodiazepine Dependence. *Journal of Substance Abuse Treatment* 1991; 8:53–59.

———. Guidelines for the Prevention of Treatment of Benzodiazepine Dependence: Summary of a Report from the Mental Health Foundation. *Addiction* 1993; 88:1707–1708.

Lader, M., and Petursson, H. Abuse Liability of Anxiolytics. In *Anxiolytics: Neurochemical, Behavioral and Clinical Perspectives,* edited by Malick, J. B., Enna, S. J., and Yamamura, H. I. 1983b Raven Press New York.

Lader, M., and Petursson, H. Long-Term Effects of Benzodiazepines. *Neuropharmacology* 1983c 22(4):527–533.

Lader, M., Ron, M., and Petursson, H. Computed Axial Brain Tomography in Long-Term Benzodiazepine Users. *Psychological Medicine* 1984b; 14:203–206.

Ladewig, D. Dependence Liability of the Benzodiazepines. *Drug and Alcohol Dependence,* 1984; 13:139–149.

Laegreid, L., Olegard, R., Conradi, N., Hagberg, G., Wahlstrom, J., and Abrahamsson, L. Congenital Malformations and Maternal Consumption of Benzodiazepines: A Case-Control Study. *Developmental Medicine and Child Neurology* 1990; 32:432–441.

Last, C. G., Hersen, M., Kazdin, A., Orvaschel, H., and Perrin, S. Anxiety Disorders in Children and Their Families. *Archives of General Psychiatry* 1991; 348:928–934.

Laughren, T. P., Battey, Y., Greenblatt, D. J., Harrop, D. S. A Controlled Trial of Diazepam Withdrawal in Chronically Anxious Outpatients. *Acta Psychiatricia Scandinavica* 1982; 65:171–179.

Lee, K. A., Vaillant, G. E., Torrey, W. C., Elder, G. H. A 50-Year Prospective Study of the Psychological Sequelae of World War II Combat. *American Journal of Psychiatry* 1995; 152:516–522.

Life magazine 1956; 41(26) p. 115.

Lin, S. C., Morse, R. M., Finlayson, R. E., and Palmen, M. A. Abuse of Benzodiazepines. Letter in *Journal of the American Medical Society* 1989; 261(20):2956–2957.

Lipman-Blumen, J. *Gender Roles and Power.* Prentice-Hall 1984 Englewood Cliffs, NJ.

Maccoby, E. E., Jacklin, C. N. *The Psychology of Sex Differences.* Stanford University Press 1974 Stanford, CA.

Macdonald, J. B. The Role of Drugs in Falls in the Elderly. *Clinics in Geriatric Medicine.* 1985: 1(3):621–636.

Marks, I. M. *Fears, Phobias, and Rituals: Panic, Anxiety and Their Disorders.* Oxford University Press 1987 New York.

Marks, I. M., de Albuquerque, A., Cottraux, J., et. al. The "Efficacy" of Alprazolam in Panic Disorder and Agoraphobia: A Critique of Recent Reports. *Archives of General Psychiatry* 1989; 46:668–669.

Marks, I. M., Greist, J., Basoglu, M., Noshirvani, H., and O'Sullivan, G. Comment on the Second Phase of the Cross-National Collaborative Panic Study. *British Journal of Psychiatry* 1992; 160:202–205.

Marks, J. The Benzodiazepines—For Good or Evil. *Neuropsychobiology* 1983; 10:115–126.

Mavissakalian, M., and Michelson, L. Two-year Follow-Up of Exposure and Imipramine Treatment of Agoraphobia. *American Journal of Psychiatry* 1986; 143:1106–1112.

Mazza, D. L., Martin, D., Spacavento, L., Jacobsen, J., and Gibbs, H. Prevalence of Anxiety Disorders in Patients with Mitral Valve Prolapse. *American Journal of Psychiatry* 1986; 143:349–352.

McClusky, H. Y., Milby, J. B., Switzer, P. K., Williams, V., and Wooten, V. Efficacy of Behavioral Versus Triazolam Treatment in Persistent Sleep-Onset Insomnia. *American Journal of Psychiatry* 1991; 148:121–126.

McNutt, L. A., Coles, B., McAuliffe, T., Baird, S., Morse, D. L., Strogatz, D. S., Baron, R. C., and Eadie, J. L. Impact of Regulation on Benzodiazepine Prescribing to a Low-Income Elderly Population, New York State. *Journal of Clinical Epidemiology* 1994; 47(6):613–625.

Melander, A., Henricson, K., Stenberg, P., Lowenhielm, P., Malmvik, J., Sternebring, B., Kaij, L., and Bergdahl, U. Anxiolytic-Hypnotic Drugs: Relationships Between Prescribing, Abuse and Suicide. *Clinical Pharmacology* 1991; 41:525–529.

Mellinger, G. D., Balter, M. B., and Uhlenhuth, E. H. Prevalence and Correlates of the Long-Term Regular Use of Anxiolytics. *Journal of the American Medical Association* 1984a; 251:375–379.

―――. Anti-Anxiety Agents: Duration of Use and Characteristics of Users in the USA. *Current Medical Research and Opinion* 1984b; 8 (supplement 4):21–36.

Melton, L. J., Riggs, B. L. Epidemiology of Age-related Fractures. In: The Osteoporotic Syndrome: Detection, Prevention, and Treatment. Avioli L. V., ed. Grune and Stratton New York 1983:45–72.

Milby, J. B., Williams, V., Hall, J. N., Khuder, S., McGill, T., and Wooten, V. Effectiveness of Combined Triazolam-Behavioral Therapy for Primary Insomnia. *American Journal of Psychiatry* 1993; 150:1259–1260.

Miller, J. B. *Toward a New Psychology of Women*. Beacon Press 1976 Boston.

Miller, N. E. Learning of Visceral and Glandular Responses. *Science* 1969; 163:434–445.

Miller, N. S. Liability and Efficacy from Long-Term Use of Benzodiazepines: Documentation and Interpretation. *Psychiatric Annals* 1995; 25(3):166–173.

Miller, N. S., and Gold, M. S. Introduction—Benzodiazepines: A Major Problem. *Journal of Substance Abuse Treatment*. 1991; 8:3–7.

Milrod, B. The Continued Usefulness of Psychoanalysis in the Treatment Armamentarium for Panic Disorder. *Journal of the American Psychoanalytic Association* 1995; 43:151–162.

Milrod, B., Busch, F. N., Hollander, E., Aronson, A., Siever, A. A 23-year old Woman with Panic Disorder Treated with Psychodynamic Psychotherapy. *Journal of Psychiatry* 153:5, May 1996.

Milrod, B., Shear, M. K. Psychodynamic Treatment of Panic: Three Case Histories. *Hospital and Community Psychiatry* 1991a; 42:311–312.

———. Dynamic Treatment of Panic Disorder: A Review. *Journal of Nervous and Mental Disease* 1991b; 179:741–743.

Mohler, H., and Okada, T. The Benzodiazepine Receptor in Normal and Pathological Human Brain. *British Journal of Psychiatry*. 1978; 133:261–268.

Moodley, P., Golombok, S., Shine, P., and Lader, M. Computed Axial Brain Tomograms in Long-Term Benzodiazepine Users. *Psychiatry Research* 1993; 48:135–144.

Morabia, A., Fabre, J., and Dunand, J. P. The Influence of Patient and Physician Gender on Prescription of Psychotropic Drugs. *Journal of Clinical Epidemiology* 1992; 45(2):111–116.

Morrice, A., Iliffe, S. Advising Patients on Their Benzodiazepine Use. Letter in *British Journal of General Practice* 1990; Feb.: 83.

Muller, C. The Overmedicated Society: Forces in the Marketplace for Medical Care. *Science* 1972; 176:488–492.

Neutel, C. I. Risk of Traffic Accident Injury After a Prescription for a Benzodiazepine. *Annals of Epidemiology* 1995; 5:239–244.

New York Times 11/16/79 p. A18.

Nikaido, A. M., Ellinwood Jr., E. H., Heatherly, D. F., and Dubow, D. Differential CNS Effects of Diazepam in Elderly Adults. *Pharmacology, Biochemistry and Behavior* 1987; 27(2):273–281.

Noyes, R., Garvey, M. J., Cook, B., and Perry, P. J. Benzodiazepine Withdrawal: A Review of the Evidence. *Journal of Clinical Psychiatry* 1988; 49:382–389.

Noyes, R., Garvey, M. J., Cook, B. L., and Suelzer, M. Controlled Discontinuation of Benzodiazepine Treatment for Patients with Panic Disorder. *American Journal of Psychiatry* 1991; 148:517–523.

Noyes, R., Reich, J., Christiansen, J., Suelzer, M., Pfohl, B., and Coryell, W. A. Outcome of Panic Disorder: Relationship to Diagnostic Subtypes and Comorbidity. *Archives of General Psychiatry* 1990; 47:809–818.

Ost, L. G. A Maintenance Program for Behavioral Treatment of Anxiety Disorders. *Behaviour Research and Therapy* 1989; 27(2):123–130.

Oster, G., Huse, D. M., Adams, S. F., Imbimbo, J., and Russell, M. W. Benzodiazepine Tranquilizers and the Risk of Accidental Injury. *American Journal of Public Health* 1990; 80:1467–1470.

Otto, M. W., Gould, R. A., and Pollack, M. H. Cognitive-Behavioral Treatment of Panic Disorder: Considerations for the Treatment of Patients Over the Long Term. *Psychiatric Annals* 1994; 24(6):307–315.

Otto, M. W., Pollack, M. H., Meltzer-Brody, S., and Rosenbaum, J. F. Cognitive-Behavioral Therapy for Benzodiazepine Discontinuation in Panic Disorder Patients. *Psychopharmacology Bulletin* 1992; 28(2):123–130.

Otto, M. W., Pollack, M. H., Sachs, G. S., Reiter, S. R., Meltzer-Brody, S., and Rosenbaum, J. F. Discontinuation of Benzodiazepine Treatment: Efficacy of Cognitive-Behavioral Therapy for Patients with Panic Disorder. *American Journal of Psychiatry* 1993; 150:1485–1490.

Palinkas, L. A., Petterson, J. S., Russell, J., and Downs, M. A. Community Patterns of Psychiatric Disorders After the Exxon *Valdez* Oil Spill. *American Journal of Psychiatry* 1993; 150:1517–1523.

Paul, S. M., Marangos, P. J., Goodwin, F. K., and Skolnick, P. Brian-Specific Benzodiazepine Receptors and Putative Endogenous Benzodiazepine-Like Compounds. *Biological Psychiatry* 1980; 15(3):407–428.

Pecknold, J. C., Swinson, R. P., Kuch, K., and Lewis, C. Alprazolam in Panic Disorder and Agoraphobia: Results from a Multicenter Trial. III. Discontinuation Effects. *Archives of General Psychiatry* 1988; 45:429–436.

Perera, K. M. H., Powell, T., Jenner, F. A. Computerized Axial Tomographic Studies Following Long-Term Use of Benzodiazepines. *Psychological Medicine* 1987; 17:775–777.

Petursson, H., Lader, M. H. Withdrawal from Long-Term Benzodiazepine Treatment. *British Medical Journal* 1981; 283:643–645.

Physicians Desk Reference (PDR). Medical Economics Data Production Co. 1996 Montvale, NJ.

Pitman, R. K., van der Kolk, B. A., Orr, S. P., Greenberg, M. S. Naloxone-Reversible Analgesic Response to Combat-Related Stimuli in Posttraumatic Disorder. *Archives of General Psychiatry* 1990; 47:541–544.

Pollack, M. H., Otto, M. W., Tesar, G. E., Cohen, L. S., Meltzer-Brody, S., and Rosenbaum, J. F. Long-Term Outcome After Acute Treatment with Alprazolam or Clonazepam for Panic Disorder. *Journal of Clinical Psychopharmacology*. 1993; 13:257–263.

Pomara, N., Stanley, B., Block, R., Berchou, R. C., Stanley, M., Greenblatt,

D. J., Newton, R. E., and Gershon S. Increased Sensitivity of the Elderly to the Central Depressant Effects of Diazepam. *Journal of Clinical Psychiatry* 1985; 46:185–187.

Poser, W., Poser, S., Roscher, D., and Argyrakis, A. Do Benzodiazepines Cause Cerebral Atrophy? *Lancet* 1983; 1:715.

Post, P., Webb, W., and Robinson, B. Relationship Between Self-Concept, Anxiety and Knowledge of Alcoholism by Gender and Age Among Adult Children of Alcoholics. *Alcoholism Treatment Quarterly* 1991; 8(3):91–95.

Prather, J. E., Minkov, N. V. Prescription for Despair: Women and Psychotropics Drugs. In *Feminist Perspectives on Addictions,* N. van dan Bergh, ed. Springer Press 1991 New York.

Pribor, E. F., Dinwiddie, S. H. Psychiatric Correlates of Incest in Childhood. *American Journal of Psychiatry* 1992; 149(1):52–56.

Raft, D., Davidson, J., Toomey, T. C., Spencer, R. F., and Lewis, B. F. Inpatient and Outpatient Patterns of Psychotropic Drug Prescribing by Nonpsychiatric Physicians. *American Journal of Psychiatry* 1995; 132(12):1309–1312.

Rainey, J. M., Aleem, A., Ortiz, A., Yeragani, V., Pohl, R., Berchou, R. A Laboratory Procedure for the Induction of Flashbacks. *American Journal of Psychiatry* 1987; 144:1317–1319.

Ray, W. A., Fought, R. L., and Decker, M. D. Psychoactive Drugs and the Risk of Injurious Motor Vehicle Crashes in Elderly Drivers. *American Journal of Epidemiology* 1992; 136(7):873–883.

Ray, W. A., Griffin, M. R., Schaffner, W., Baugh, D. K., and Melton, J. Psychotropic Drug Use and the Risk of Hip Fracture. *New England Journal of Medicine* 1987; 316:363–369.

Reidenberg, M. M. Effect of the Requirement of Triplicate Prescriptions for Benzodiazepines in New York State. *Clin Pharmacol Ther* 1991; 50(2):129–131.

Rickels, K., Case, W. G., Downing, R. W., and Fridman, R. B. One-Year Follow-Up of Anxious Patients Treated with Diazepam. *Journal of Clinical Pharmacology* 1986a; 6(1):32–36.

Rickels, D., Case, W. G., Downing, R. W., and Winokur, A. Long-Term Diazepam Therapy and Clinical Outcome. *Journal of the American Medical Association* 1983; 250:767–771.

Rickels, K., Case, W. G., Schweizer, E., Garcia-Espana, F., and Fridman, R. B. Long-Term Benzodiazepine Users 3 Years After Participation in a Discontinuation Program. *American Journal of Psychiatry.* 1991; 148:757–761.

Rickels, K., Case, W. G., Schweizer, E., Swenson, C., and Fridman, R. B. Low-Dose Dependence in Chronic Benzodiazepine Users: A Preliminary Report on 119 patients. *Psychopharmacology Bulletin* 1986b 22(2):407–415.

Rickels, K., Case, W. G., Winokur, A., and Swenson, C. Long-Term Benzodiazepine Therapy: Benefits and Risks. *Psychopharmacology Bulletin* 1984 20(4):608–615.

Rickels, K., and Clyde, D. J. Clyde Mood Scale Changes in Anxious Outpatients Produced by Chlordiazepoxide Therapy. *Journal of Nervous and Mental Disease* 1967 145:154–157.

Rickels, K., Schweizer, E., Case, W. G., and Greenblatt, D. J. Long-Term Therapeutic use of Benzodiazepines. *Archives of General Psychiatry* 1990; 47:899–907.

Rickels, K., Schweizer, E., Csanalosi, I., Case, W. G., and Chung, H. Long-Term Treatment of Anxiety and Risk of Withdrawal. *Archives of General Psychiatry* 1988; 45:444–450.

Rickels, K., Schweizer, E., Weiss, S., Zavodnik, S. Maintenance Drug Treatment for Panic Disorder. *Archives of General Psychiatry* 1993; 50:61–68.

Rodrigo, E. K., King, M. B., Williams, P. Health of Long-Term Benzodiazepine Users. *British Medical Journal* 1988; 296:603–606.

Romach, M., Busto, U., Somer, G., Kaplan, H. L., and Sellers, E. Clinical Aspects of Chronic Use of Alprazolam and Lorazepam. *American Journal of Psychiatry* 1995; 152:1161–1167.

Rosenbaum, J. F., Biederman, J., Gersten, M., Hirshfeld, D. R., Meminger, S. R., Herman, J. B., Kagan, J., Reznick, J. S., and Snidman, N. Behavioral Inhibition in Children of Parents with Panic Disorder and Agoraphobia. *Archives of General Psychiatry* 1988; 45:463–470.

Rosenbaum, J. F., Biederman, J., Bolduc, E. A., Hirshfeld, D. R., Faraone, S. V., and Kagan, J. Comorbidity of Parental Anxiety Disorders as Risk for Childhood-Onset Anxiety in Inhibited Children. *American Journal of Psychiatry* 1992; 149:475–481.

Ross, H. E. Benzodiazepine Use and Anxiolytic Abuse and Dependence in Treated Alcoholics. *Addiction* 1993; 88:209–218.

Roy-Byrne, P., Geraci, M., and Uhde, T. W. Life Events and the Onset of Panic Disorder. *American Journal of Psychiatry* 1986; 143:1424–1427.

Roy-Byrne, P., Dager, S. E., Cowley, D. S., Vitaliano, P., and Dunner, D. L. Relapse and Rebound Following Discontinuation of Benzodiazepine Treatment of Panic Attacks: Alprazolam Verus Diazepam. *American Journal of Psychiatry* 1989: 146:860–865.

Russell, D. *Sexual Exploitation: Rape, Child Sexual Abuse, and Workplace Harassment.* Sage Publications 1984 Beverly Hills, California.

Salzman, C. Benzodiazepine Treatment of Panic and Agoraphobic Symptoms: Use, Dependence, Toxicity, Abuse. *J Psychiatric Research* 1993; 27(supplement 1):97–110.

Schatzberg, A. F. Overview of Anxiety Disorders: Prevalence, Biology, Course and Treatment. *Journal of Clinical Psychiatry* 1991; 52(supplement 7):5–9.

Schmauss, C., and Krieg, J. C. Enlargement of Cerebrospinal Fluid Spaces in Long-Term Benzodiazepine Abusers. *Psychological Medicine* 1987; 17:869–873.

Schneider-Helmert, D. Why Low-Dose Benzodiazepine-Dependent Insomniacs Can't Escape Their Sleeping Pills. *Acta Psychiatricia Scandinavica* 1988; 78:706–711.

Schopf, J. Withdrawal Phenomena after Long-Term Administration of

Benzodiazepines. A Review of Recent Investigations. *Pharmacopsychiatry* 1983; 16:1–8.

Schweizer, E., Rickels, K., Weiss, S., and Zavodnick, S. Maintenance Drug Treatment for Panic Disorder. *Archives of General Psychiatry* 1993; 50:51–60.

Serfaty, M., and Masterton, G. Fatal Poisonings Attributed to Benzodiazepines in Britain During the 1980s. *British Journal of Psychiatry* 1993; 163:386–393.

Shapiro, A. K., Struening, E. L., Shapiro, E., and Milcarek, B. I. Diazepam: How Much Better Than Placebo? *J Psychiat Res* 1983; 17(1):51–73.

Shear, M. K., Cooper, A. M., Klerman, G. L., Busch, F. N., Shapiro, T. A Psychodynamic Model of Panic Disorder. *American Journal of Psychiatry* 1993; 150:859–866.

Shear, M. K., Pilkonis, P. A., Cloitre, M., and Leon, A. C. Cognitive Behavioral Treatment Compared with Nonprescriptive Treatment of Panic Disorder. *Archives of General Psychiatry* 1994; 51:395–401.

Sheehan, D. V. *The Anxiety Disease*. Bantam Books 1986 New York.

Shore, J. H., Tatum, E. L., Vollmer, W. M. Psychiatric Reactions to Disaster. *American Journal of Psychiatry* 1986; 143:590–595.

Silove, D., Manicavasagar, V., O'Connell, D., Morris-Yates, A. Genetic factors in Early Separation Anxiety: Implications for the Genesis of Adult Anxiety Disorders. *Acta Psychiatricia Scandinavica* 1995; 92:17–24.

Simpson, R. J., Power, K. G., and Swanson, V. Age-Band Prevalence Rates of Long-Term Benzodiazepine Users. *British Journal of General Practice* 1990; 4:168–169.

Skre, I., Onstad, S., Edvardsen, J., Torgersen, S., Kringlen, E. A Family Study of Anxiety Disorders: Familial Transmission and Relationship to Mood Disorder and Psychoactive Substance Use Disorder. *Acta Psychiatricia Scandinavica* 1994; 90:366–374.

Snyder, S. H. Benzodiazepine Receptors. *Psychiatric Annals* Nov. 11, 1981:19–23.

Solomon, K., and Hart, R. Pitfalls and Prospects in Clinical Research on Antianxiety Drugs: Benzodiazepines and Placebo—A Research Review. *Journal of Clinical Psychiatry* 1978 39:823–831.

Southwick, S. M., Krystal, J. H., Morgan, A., Johnson, D., Nagy, L. M., Nicolaou, A., Heninger, G. R., Charney, D. S. Abnormal Noradrenergic Function in Posttraumatic Stress Disorder. *Archives of General Psychiatry* 1993; 50:266–274.

Spiegel, D. A., Bruce, T. J., Gregg, S. F., and Nuzzarello, A. Does Cognitive Behavior Therapy Assist Slow-Taper Alprazolam Discontinuation in Panic Disorders? *American Journal of Psychiatry* 1994; 151:876–881.

Stein, M. B., Walker, J. R., Anderson, G., Hazen, A. L., Ross, C. A., Eldridge, G., Forde, D. R. Childhood Physical and Sexual Abuse in Patients with Anxiety Disorders and in a Community Sample. *American Journal of Psychiatry* 1996; 153:275–277.

Summers, R. S., Schlutte, A., and Summers, B. Benzodiazepine Use in a Small Community Hospital. *S Afr Med J* 1990; 78:721–725.

Tallman, J. F., Paul, S. M., Skolnick, P., and Gallager, D. W. Receptors for the Age of Anxiety: Pharmacology of the Benzodiazepines. *Science* 1980; 207(Jan):274–281.

Taylor, C. B. and Arnow, B. *The Nature and Treatment of Anxiety Disorders.* Macmillan, The Free Press 1988 New York.

Thomson, M., and Smith, W. A. Prescribing Benzodiazepines for Noninstitutionalized Elderly, *Canadian Family Physician* 1995; 41:792–798.

Tinetti, M. E., Speechley, M., and Ginter, S. F. Risk Factors for Falls Among Elderly Persons Living in the Community. *New England Journal of Medicine* 1988; 319:1701-1707.

Tobin, J. M., Lorenz, A. A., Brousseau, E. R., et al: Clinical Evaluation of Oxazepam for the Management of Anxiety. *Diseases of the Nervous System* 1964; 25:589–696.

Torgersen, S. Genetic Factors in Anxiety Disorders. *Archives of General Psychiatry* 1983; 40:1085–1089.

Tyrer, P., Murphy, S., Kingdon, D., Brothwell, J., Gregory, S., Seivewright, N., Ferguson, B., Barczak, P., Darling, C., and Johnson, A. L. The Nottingham Study of Neurotic Disorder: Comparison of Drug and Psychological Treatments. *Lancet* 1988; July 30:235–240.

Uhde, T. W., and Kellner, C. H. Cerebral Ventricular Size in Panic Disorder. *Journal of Affective Disorders* 1987; 12:175–178.

Wall Street Journal. Managed Care's Focus on Psychiaric Drugs Alarms Many Doctors. Dec. 1, 95, p. 1.

Wallerstein, J. S., and Berlin, K. J. Surviving the Breakup: How Children and Parents Cope with Divorce. Basic Books 1980 New York.

Wallerstein, J. S., and Blakeslee, S. *Second Chances: Men, Women, and Children a Decade After Divorce.* Ticknor and Fields 1989 New York.

Webb, W., Post, P., Robinson, B., and Moreland, L. Self-Concept, Anxiety, and Knowledge Exhibited by Adult Children of Alcoholics and Adult Children of Nonalcoholics. *Journal of Alcohol and Drug Education* 1992; (38)106–114.

Weintraub, M., Singh, S., Byrne, L., Maharaj, K., and Guttmacher, L. Consequences of the 1989 New York Triplicate Benzodiazepine Prescription Regulations. *Journal of the American Medical Association* 1991; 266:2392–2397.

Weyerer, S., Dilling, H. Psychiatric and Physical Illness, Sociodemographic Characteristics, and the Use of Psychotropic Drugs in the Community: Results from the Upper Bavarian Field Study. *Journal of Clinical Epidemiology* 1991; 44:303–311.

Wiseman, S. M., Spencer-Peet, J. Prescribing for Alcoholics. A Survey of Drugs Taken Prior to Admission to an Alcoholism Unit. *The Practitioner* 1985; 229:88–89.

Wolpe, J. *The Practice of Behavior Therapy.* Pergamon Press. 1973 New York.

Woods, J. H., Katz, J. L. and Winger, G. Abuse Liability of Benzodiazepines. *Pharmacological Reviews* 1987; 39(4):251–413.

INDEX